THE BEGINNER'S GUIDE TO UNDERSTANDING SCHIZOPHRENIA

All the latest on symptoms, causes, and treatment in plain language for people in a hurry

Dr. Hayden Finch

Copyright © 2020 by Hayden C. Finch, PhD

All rights reserved. No part of this book may be reproduced or used in any manner without written permission of the copyright owner.

First edition January 2020

Contents

INTRODUCTION 1

PART I: Clinical Manifestation.. 2

Chapter 1: Diagnostic Criteria & Symptom Categories 3

Chapter 2: Clinical Course 13

Chapter 3: Sex Differences 16

Chapter 4: Schizophrenia as a Spectrum... 19

Chapter 5: Relationship to Other Psychotic Disorders 21

Chapter 6: Co-Occurring Conditions 27

Chapter 7: Violence 32

Chapter 8: Insight 34

PART II: Causes, Risk Factors, & Pathophysiology..35

Chapter 9: Early Explanations 36

Chapter 10: Risk Factors 38

Chapter 11: Neuroanatomy 45

Chapter 12: Neurophysiology 47

Chapter 13: Neurodevelopment... 51

Chapter 14: Viral & Immunological Theory... 55

PART III: Treatment..56

Chapter 15: Medical Model vs. Psychiatric Rehabilitation 57

Chapter 16: Treatment Planning 59

Chapter 17: Biological Treatments 65

Chapter 18: Psychosocial Treatments 69

Chapter 19: Inpatient Services..80

SUMMARY..82

REFERENCES 85

INTRODUCTION

Psychotic disorders can be baffling. It's certainly not something we're taught about in school, and it's hard to know what information on television or the internet is accurate. The objective of this book is to provide you with practical guidance in understanding schizophrenia. In the first part, we'll review the definition of schizophrenia; provide examples of the most common symptoms; detail its relationship to other psychotic disorders; and discuss the most common co-occurring conditions. In the second part, we'll talk about historical and current understandings of what causes schizophrenia; review the risk factors for schizophrenia; and discuss how schizophrenia impacts the brain and the person more globally -- this is where we'll talk about genetics, neuroanatomy, neurophysiology, neurodevelopment, and substance use. Finally, in the third part, we'll talk about evidence-based treatment approaches to schizophrenia, beginning with a discussion of different treatment models and then reviewing how treatment plans are developed before finally discussing a host of interventions, including medication, skills training, psychotherapy, and family interventions.

By the end of this book, you'll be able to:

- Distinguish between positive and negative psychotic symptoms
- Identify the major mental health conditions that co-occur with schizophrenia
- Name at least two factors that increase risk for schizophrenia
- Explain how cannabis use affects risk for schizophrenia
- Describe the recovery model of schizophrenia
- Identify the major classes of medication effective in treating schizophrenia
- Explain the importance of family support in treating a person with schizophrenia

Sounds like a lot, right? But soon, you'll know it all.

PART I

Clinical Manifestation

Schizophrenia is a complex condition that is poorly understood by the general public and even by many mental health clinicians, who receive little training on the condition. But it's important to understand because it's the most debilitating and costly of all adult psychiatric illnesses (Combs & Mueser, 2007). In fact, it has been estimated to be one of the top 10 most disabling conditions in the world (reviewed in Combs & Mueser, 2007). This guide will cover the information necessary to (1) effectively identify people in your life who might have schizophrenia and (2) find the support you need as a person with schizophrenia, support person of a person with schizophrenia, or curious lay person.

Chapter 1

Diagnostic Criteria & Symptom Categories

See, here's the thing. We treat mental health diagnosis like medical diagnoses, but they're different. In medicine, diagnostic criteria represent known biological pathologies. For example, tuberculosis is diagnosed when we figure out that a person has been infected specifically with mycobacterium tuberculosis -- if any other bacterium or pathogen is the culprit, it's not tuberculosis, and another diagnosis would be made. But it's different in mental health. Diagnostic criteria in mental health don't necessarily follow known biological pathologies; instead, they follow expert opinion (at least for now...we hope that changes one day). A while back, a group of people literally just sat down and made a list of symptoms and labeled them as disorders. And because of that, mental health diagnosis isn't necessarily all that accurate or helpful. We'll discuss that more in Chapter 4, but for now, to understand what schizophrenia is, a simple review of the expert consensus will suffice.

One thing that points to the validity issues of diagnosis based on expert opinion is that we essentially have two different definitions of schizophrenia. Mental health providers use two different manuals to know what the symptoms of schizophrenia are. One is called the Diagnostic and Statistical Manual of Mental Disorders (or DSM-5) and the other is called the International Classification of Diseases (or ICD-10).

To understand the symptoms of schizophrenia, let's start with the DSM-5. Because a lot of these terms and symptoms might be new to you, we'll chat more about what they mean. But first, let's just get the criteria outlined.

DSM Criteria

According to the DSM-5 (2013), schizophrenia is diagnosed when the following six conditions are met:

1. The person has at least two of the following symptoms for a significant portion of time during a *one-month* period:

    a. Delusions

    b. Hallucinations

    c. Disorganized speech

    d. Grossly disorganized or catatonic behavior

    e. Negative symptoms

    At least one of the symptoms must be hallucinations, delusions, or disorganized speech. When these symptoms are present, this is called the *acute phase* of the illness.

AND

2. For a significant portion of time, the person's ability to function at work, in their relationships, or in taking care of themselves, must be *markedly below* their *prior* level of functioning.

AND

3. The person must have had continuous *signs* of the illness for at least *six* months, including at least *one* month where the symptoms listed above were active. This six months can include periods when the symptoms aren't as severe as you'd typically see in the acute phase. The person may only experience negative symptoms during this period or they might have symptoms in a less severe form. For example, rather than paranoia, they might have odd beliefs; or rather than hallucinations, they might have odd perceptual experiences. So six months of those milder symptoms plus at least one month of full-blown psychotic symptoms.

AND

4. Other related disorders (e.g., schizoaffective disorder, depression with psychotic features, bipolar disorder with psychotic features) have been ruled out. If the person has major depressive or manic episodes, they either don't occur during the acute phase of the illness or, if they do occur during the acute phase, they're present for a minority of the time.

AND

5. The symptoms aren't related to substance use or a medical condition.

AND

6. If the person also has a history of autism or a communication disorder with onset in childhood, schizophrenia is only added as a diagnosis if prominent delusions or hallucinations (plus the other required symptoms of schizophrenia) are present for at least one month.

So you see, diagnosis isn't as simple as determining that a person has certain typical signs and symptoms of schizophrenia. We also have to (1) rule out other potential causes of those signs and symptoms, (2) note how difficult it is for the person to function in everyday life, and (3) examine how their ability to function has changed over time.

ICD-10 Criteria

According to the ICD-10 (1992), there are no strictly "pathognomonic symptoms" of schizophrenia. That's a fancy word meaning there are no symptoms that are specifically and uniquely indicative of schizophrenia -- the symptoms also exist in other conditions. However, the "normal requirement" is the following:

1. At least one very clear of the following symptoms, or two or more symptoms if they are less clear-cut, has been present for most of the time during *one month* or more:

    a. The belief that your thoughts are being echoed, that someone or something is inserting thoughts in your head or withdrawing thoughts from your head, or that your thoughts are being broadcast out loud

    b. Delusions that your mind, body, thoughts, actions, or sensations are being controlled, influenced, or obstructed by an outside force or entity

    c. Hearing voices that give a running commentary on your behavior or discuss you amongst themselves; or hearing other voices coming from some part of your body

    d. Various other delusions that are completely impossible, like thinking you're some sort of important religious or political figure or that you have superhuman powers and abilities

OR

2. At least two of the following have been clearly present for most of the time during *one month* or more:

    a. Any type of hallucinations that either (1) are accompanied by fleeting or half-formed delusions or (2) occur every day for weeks or months on end

    b. Incoherent or irrelevant speech or made-up words

    c. Catatonic behavior (more on that later)

    d. Negative symptoms that clearly aren't related to depression or medication side effects

    e. A significant and consistent change in the person's overall behavior, such as loss of interest, aimlessness, idleness, self-absorbed attitude, or social withdrawal

Those are the criteria. But because these symptoms aren't symptoms you typically see in your friends (even the ones who are open about their mental health) and a lot of the terms might be new to you, let's discuss some examples of these symptoms.

The symptoms of schizophrenia are typically organized into three categories (Shevlin, Mcelroy, Bentall, Reininghaus, & Murphy, 2016): positive symptoms, negative symptoms, and disorganized symptoms.

Positive Symptoms

Despite urges to think of positive symptoms as "good" or "constructive" symptoms, "positive" in this case means there is an experience that is *added* to what is typical.

Positive = Present rather than absent, as normal

For example, the *absence* of hallucinations is typical, so if a person is hearing voices, that is something that is *present* that should not be. Delusions also fall in this category because unusual beliefs about self, others, or the world are added to the usual experience.

Hallucinations are the experience of a real sensory event despite there being no external stimuli causing that perception. For example, auditory hallucinations involve having the experience of really hearing something (e.g., a voice, music, bells, whispers, buzzing sounds, muffled voices) despite there being no actual sound in the environment. While most of us can distinguish between a song that is stuck in our head and a song we are actually hearing, this distinction can be much more difficult for a person with schizophrenia to make. Songs are rarely distressing, but imagine if you couldn't tell whether the critical and demanding thoughts in your head were your own self-talk or if they were coming from someone else. Believing that what you're hearing is coming from outside of you can be frightening.

About 75% of people with schizophrenia report hallucinations, with auditory hallucinations being the most common form (reviewed in Combs & Mueser, 2007). Auditory hallucinations can be continuous or intermittent. Most often, the voices heard by a person with schizophrenia are derogatory, critical, or abusive, though some can be friendly (reviewed in Combs & Mueser, 2007). Under the ICD-10 criteria above, it was mentioned that some people with schizophrenia hear voices that give a running commentary on the person's behavior or hear multiple voices having a conversation; this is an uncommon experience but seems to be very specific to schizophrenia (reviewed in Combs & Mueser, 2007). Historically, visual hallucinations were thought to be rare in schizophrenia, but more recent evidence suggests this may have been inaccurate (reviewed in Combs & Mueser, 2007). Most often, visual hallucinations reported in schizophrenia involve perceptions of shadows, ghosts, or figures or seeing the walls moving or the floor moving.

Delusions are beliefs that are firmly held despite being contradicted by reality or logical argument. In schizophrenia, delusions can take essentially any form, though the most common are persecutory delusions. Persecutory delusions are beliefs that a certain person, group, or entity (e.g., the FBI) has clear intentions to harm the person with schizophrenia. Other common delusions are beliefs that you're being controlled by aliens, that you're receiving special messages through the television or other media, that you're an important religious figure, that you have powers (e.g., to control the weather, to communicate with aliens), or that you have something seriously wrong with your body (e.g., like you got run over by a bus but are still alive).

Positive symptoms tend to fluctuate over the course of the illness and go into remission at times.

Negative Symptoms

If positive symptoms mean something is present that shouldn't be, negative symptoms mean something is missing that *should* be there.

Negative = *Not* Present, when normally it is

For example, it is typical for people to experience a variety of emotions and facial expressions. So if a person is feeling very flat, uses very few words, or is socially withdrawn, those are symptoms that are missing from the typical experience. Other examples of negative symptoms include the inability to experience pleasure, slowed speech, physical inertia, and apathy. Apathy is a major problem for a lot of people with schizophrenia, and they often lack interest or motivation in anything, including speaking to people.

You might be thinking that sounds like depression, and negative symptoms are frequently confused with depression. The difference is that negative symptoms aren't associated with sadness -- you just see the lack of interest, slowed down behavior, and withdrawal without the emotional experience of depression. Not only do people with schizophrenia often have no emotional expression, but sometimes they'll show inappropriate emotions, like laughing at strange times, which can obviously impact how well they get along with other people. Negative symptoms don't get nearly as much attention as positive symptoms, but they're really important to pay attention to because people who experience severe negative symptoms are much more likely to have difficulty functioning in their everyday lives (Campellone, Sanchez, & Kring, 2016).

Whereas positive symptoms tend to fluctuate over the course of the illness and go into remission at times, negative symptoms are much more constant and pervasive (reviewed in Combs & Mueser, 2007).

Disorganized Symptoms

There's also a group of symptoms called "disorganized symptoms." These symptoms represent a fragmentation of behavior and experience. In other words, when information isn't coordinated or integrated well, illogical thoughts and speech and purposeless motor activity can develop. So people with schizophrenia can have major difficulty keeping their train of thought, which can then make it difficult to understand what they're saying. They sometimes speak incoherently, respond to questions with unrelated answers, shift topics abruptly without any apparent connection between topics, or drift to different topics before coming back around to the topic at hand a while later. They even can make up words, rhyme words randomly, and get stuck repeating words or phrases.

Just like a person with schizophrenia might have difficulty expressing a complete thought coherently, they can also have difficulty completing a task or behavior in a meaningful way. This means they might have unpredictable or inappropriate emotional reactions, engage in bizarre or seemingly purposeless behavior (e.g., wearing multiple layers of clothes; maintaining peculiar postures for no apparent reason), or see a major decline in their general functioning (like with grooming and hygiene tasks, for example). At the extreme, we can see interesting symptoms such as "waxy flexibility," which is when a person will leave their limbs in a position another person puts them in, as if they're made out of clay. We can even see complete immobility or stupor.

Cognitive Impairments

So those are the three symptom categories. In addition to these specific symptoms, many people with schizophrenia experience major cognitive deficits, or problems in how they process information. Although cognitive impairments aren't technically "symptoms" of schizophrenia, they're such a core part of the symptom presentation that they could reasonably be considered symptoms. People with schizophrenia perform consistently and significantly lower than people without schizophrenia on almost all cognitive tasks (reviewed in Combs & Mueser, 2007). Their deficits include problems setting and working toward goals (Poppe et al., 2016), temporarily holding information in mind for processing (Gold et al., 2017), and general executive functioning. Executive functioning is a set of advanced cognitive skills that helps us gather information from the environment, structure it so we can evaluate it, and change our behavior in response to what is happening in our environment. This includes things like planning ahead, paying attention, switching focus, organizing and managing time and materials, remembering details, inhibiting inappropriate behavior, and multitasking. Because such a wide range of related skills are impaired in schizophrenia, it's not clear whether there are isolated skill impairments or whether a more generalized impairment is responsible for the whole range of deficits (reviewed in Gold et al., 2017).

Beyond executive functioning, individuals with schizophrenia also tend to be able to process less information, they process it more slowly, they show deficits in attention and short-term memory, they have trouble understanding concepts, and they have difficulty keeping track of their thoughts (reviewed in Combs & Mueser, 2007, and Silverstein, Spaulding, & Menditto, 2006). These cognitive deficits are seen in children at high risk for developing schizophrenia as well as people experiencing their first psychotic episode, people who are medicated and unmedicated, and people in remission from the acute symptoms (reviewed in Combs & Mueser, 2007). This points to how pervasive these cognitive deficits are and how important they are in the schizophrenia clinical picture. Importantly, all these deficits in thinking skills are separate from the person's intelligence. Schizophrenia does *not* impair intellectual functioning, but it does impair attention and other cognitive processes (reviewed in Combs & Mueser, 2007).

Accompanying these deficits in how *well* people with schizophrenia process information are biases in *how* they process information. In the early stages of the condition, people respond differently to information in the environment, which can affect development of schizophrenia. For example, people who are developing schizophrenia tend to be more sensitive to stress, their brains get overwhelmed because they're identifying certain stimuli that are irrelevant as important, and they chronically feel threatened because they keep anticipating bad events in their lives (Reininghaus et al., 2016). The experience whereby their brains misinterpret random experiences as important is thought to create psychotic symptoms (Reininghaus et al., 2016). For example, if your brain decides some sort of random, aberrant sound isn't random but is actually meaningful and important, this can be experienced as an auditory hallucination.

People with schizophrenia also have deficits in how they process social information, which has important implications for how they function socially. These cognitive deficits are independent of the deficits they have in processing other types of information and are governed by different brain processes (reviewed in Combs & Mueser, 2007). We'll chat more about social cognition in Chapter 18.

Associated Features

In early adulthood, most people are achieving important developmental milestones in occupational, educational, and social functioning. But this is when schizophrenia tends to set in. Unsurprisingly, then, individuals with schizophrenia often fail to meet these milestones. They are less likely to be married and are less likely to remain married (reviewed in Combs & Mueser, 2007). They are also less likely to complete higher education and are more likely to live in poverty. We don't know exactly how or why schizophrenia is related to socioeconomic status. One hypothesis is that people with schizophrenia have disabilities that affect their ability to sustain employment, which increases risk for poverty (reviewed in Combs & Mueser, 2007). Another is that if they were raised in poverty, the associated stress could actually make them more likely to develop schizophrenia (reviewed in Combs & Mueser, 2007). We'll chat more about how stress affects risk for schizophrenia in Chapter 10.

Now that you know the symptoms of schizophrenia and some of the other features associated with it, let's move into how it changes over the lifespan.

Chapter 2

Clinical Course

The most obvious symptoms of schizophrenia tend to show up for the first time in the late teens and early 20s, between ages 16 and 25. But more subtle signs and markers for the condition are often present long before that, which we'll chat more about later. Childhood-onset schizophrenia is thought to be an entirely different condition than adolescent- or adult-onset schizophrenia (reviewed in Combs & Mueser, 2007). It's more common (but still really rare) to develop schizophrenia after age 40 than it is to develop it in childhood. About 23% of people with schizophrenia experience their first episode after age 40. These people usually have better social, educational, and occupational functioning than people who have the typical onset in late adolescence and early adulthood, and they usually have more positive symptoms and fewer negative and disorganized symptoms than is typical (reviewed in Combs & Mueser, 2007).

The "acute" phase of schizophrenia is when the hallucinations and delusions show up and major functional decline sets in. This is preceded by a period of months to years of "prodromal symptoms," often during late adolescence. Social isolation and bizarre or suspicious thoughts in this period of development can increase risk for schizophrenia, especially if there's also a family history of schizophrenia (Lambert & Kinsley, 2011). Someone is at "clinical high risk" for schizophrenia if they possess a certain number of risk factors (see Chapter 10). Some of those individuals will ultimately develop schizophrenia, while others won't. Currently, it's very difficult to distinguish people who are actually experiencing the onset of a psychotic condition from people who are at "clinical high risk" but aren't actually going to go on to develop a psychotic condition (Schmidt et al., 2016). Even though it's hard to tell them apart, a decline in social functioning in adolescence is a particularly effective predictor of which high risk individuals will ultimately develop schizophrenia (Carrión et al.,

2018). Accurate prediction is important because the length of time the illness is left untreated (e.g., at the beginning stages of development of schizophrenia) is a powerful indicator of how well the person does in the long term. That's why early detection is a focus of many interventions for individuals experiencing their first psychotic episode (Oliver et al. 2018).

During the prodromal period, subtle signs and markers of schizophrenia gradually increase in intensity. The prodromal symptoms don't meet criteria for schizophrenia during this period, but people who know the individual begin to notice changes in the person. This includes disruptions in sleep, anxiety, depression, irritability, paranoia, and odd beliefs as well as changes in how they're functioning at school, at work, and in their relationships (reviewed in Combs & Mueser, 2007).

The prodromal period can last anywhere from several days to as long as five years (reviewed in Combs & Mueser, 2007). During that time, there may be gradual or extremely rapid changes in how the person functions, with folks experiencing the rapid onset having a somewhat better prognosis in the long term (reviewed in Combs & Mueser, 2007). The prodromal period is followed by the first psychotic episode, which is the period when the classic symptoms of schizophrenia first present. Early intervention during this period is critical and can change the entire lifetime course of the disorder.

There's considerable variation in how schizophrenia is experienced from person to person, and even across a single person's lifetime. But most often the symptoms come and go. Periods when the person experiences more severe symptoms (called acute episodes, or relapses) alternate with periods when the symptoms more or less go away (called remission). Even during remission, though, most people don't return to the same level of functioning they had before they developed schizophrenia (reviewed in Combs & Mueser, 2007). The goal of treatment is often to prevent or minimize the frequency or severity of relapses. This is in part because each relapse makes future symptoms more persistent and causes more impairment in how the person thinks and how they function in their life (reviewed in Combs & Mueser, 2007).

Given the severity of the illness, the prognosis for schizophrenia is usually considered poor to fair (reviewed in Combs & Mueser, 2007). However, effective treatments exist that can result in symptom remission and recovery, which we'll discuss more in Part III.

Chapter 3

Sex Differences

There are *not* known to be major sex differences in schizophrenia in terms of family history of psychotic disorders, birth complications, minor physical anomalies (see below), or neurological soft signs (see below) (Leung & Chue, 2000), but there may be some differences between men and women with schizophrenia in how the brain works in specific areas (Shahab et al., 2017). And there are significant differences between men and women diagnosed with schizophrenia (Leung & Chue, 2000) in how common the diagnosis is, when it starts, how it manifests, the response to treatment, and the overall prognosis.

Incidence

Schizophrenia is experienced by between 0.3% and 0.7% of the world population, which represents over 2 million Americans. It's remarkably stable across different populations and cultures (reviewed in Combs & Mueser, 2007), but men tend to be diagnosed with schizophrenia 1.4 times more often than women (Mcgrath et al., 2004). This means for every 10 women diagnosed, 14 men are diagnosed.

Age of Onset

Men tend to experience the first symptoms about five years earlier than women (Loranger, 1984), with the average age of onset being around age 21 for men and around age 27 for women (Lambert & Kinsley, 2011). Men who are ultimately diagnosed with schizophrenia begin experiencing psychotic symptoms by age 30 90% of the time, whereas 66% of women who are ultimately diagnosed with schizophrenia begin experiencing psychotic symptoms by age 30. And while 17% of women experience their first symptoms after age 35 and 10% of women show no signs of psychosis until after age 40, only 2% of men show their first symptoms after age 35. That was confusing. Here's a table.

	Average Age of Onset	Onset by Age 30	Onset After Age 35
Men	21	90%	2%
Women	27	66%	17%

Clinical Manifestation

Men show more negative symptoms (inability to experience pleasure, slowed speech, physical inertia, apathy) and cognitive deficits (difficulty solving problems and processing information) and they have more abnormalities in how their brains are built and how they work (Leung & Chue, 2000). By contrast, women tend to show more emotional symptoms (e.g., depression, anxiety), auditory hallucinations, and persecutory delusions.

Treatment Response

Women tend to respond better to antipsychotic medications than men (at least prior to menopause), but they have more side effects (Leung & Chue, 2000). Interestingly, some research suggests social skills training may be more helpful for men than women (reviewed in Combs & Mueser, 2007), but we don't know why this is. Also, women with schizophrenia have different treatment needs than men, in part because they manifest the illness differently but also because they function differently. Women are more likely than men to get married and have children, so they have more needs related to intimate relationships, family planning, and parenting than men do (reviewed in Combs & Mueser, 2007).

Prognosis

Women tend to have a more favorable prognosis, at least in the short- and middle-term, and spend less time in the hospital than men (reviewed in Combs & Mueser, 2007). This is thought to be because they don't use drugs and alcohol as much and because they have better family support (Leung & Chue, 2000). Men often come from more critical and less supportive families, which has a negative impact on prognosis (Leung & Chue, 2000).

We don't know exactly why women with schizophrenia fare better than men. Lots of theories have been proposed, including hormonal explanations about how estrogen interacts with dopamine, how women cope with stress, and how much social support they have, but none of these theories has received much support (reviewed in Combs & Mueser, 2007).

Chapter 4

Schizophrenia as a Spectrum

As mentioned earlier in the ICD-10 symptom review (Chapter 1), none of the symptoms of schizophrenia are unique to the diagnosis. All are seen in many other conditions.

For example, hallucinations are seen in psychotic disorders as well as mood disorders with psychotic features (e.g., major depressive disorder with psychotic features; bipolar disorder with psychotic features) and some neurocognitive disorders (e.g., some dementias have hallucinations). The only factor that appears to distinguish hallucinations in schizophrenia from those seen in other mental health conditions is the *age of onset in late adolescence* (Waters & Fernyhough, 2016).

Similarly, paranoia can be a symptom of schizophrenia, or it can show up when a person is intoxicated with or withdrawing from drugs, or even if they have a personality disorder. This fact complicates diagnosis, especially among the psychotic disorders themselves.

In short, **the presence of any specific symptom is insufficient to diagnose schizophrenia; instead, it is important to consider how that symptom co-occurs with other symptoms and functional impairments.**

Not only are the symptoms germane to many conditions, but they also exist in the general population (Shevlin et al., 2016). For example, people in the general population hear voices and show similar brain activity during these hallucinatory experiences (Baumeister, Sedgwick, Howes, & Peters, 2017). So schizophrenia isn't a discrete disease that one "has" or doesn't "have." Instead, it's a set of *experiences* on the severe end of a spectrum or continuum of psychotic symptoms. People who experience these subclinical psychotic experiences but don't have schizophrenia are often influenced by the same risk factors that influence the prevalence of schizophrenia. And they experience similar (though much less severe) cognitive deficits (reviewed in Murray, Bhavsar, Tripoli, & Howes, 2017).

The fact that the symptoms are on a spectrum makes diagnosis relatively arbitrary. This is similar to what is seen in some medical conditions. For example, if a person's A1C levels are above 5.7% on two separate tests, they might be diagnosed with prediabetes, though this figure is relatively arbitrary. And if the levels rise above 6.5%, another arbitrary figure, then the diagnosis might be elevated to diabetes. As with blood sugar, **it's not that a person has various psychotic symptoms that results in the diagnosis; rather, when the symptoms and their associated impairment rise above a certain arbitrary threshold, a psychotic disorder diagnosis is considered**. And if the symptoms persist and are associated with other relevant factors, a diagnosis of schizophrenia may be made.

Despite these problems with diagnosis, diagnosis tends to be very stable in schizophrenia (and schizoaffective disorder and mood disorders with psychotic features), meaning that people who are accurately diagnosed with schizophrenia rarely have their diagnosis changed to another condition (Fusar-Poli et al., 2016). On the other hand, there's much less diagnostic stability with related conditions like delusional disorder, brief psychotic disorder, substance-induced psychotic disorder, and unspecified psychotic disorder; those diagnoses are most frequently changed to schizophrenia. Being able to accurately diagnose at the first sign of a psychotic illness is critical for rallying the most appropriate interventions, in part because schizophrenia has a much different treatment plan and is associated with more functional difficulties than mood disorders with psychotic features and some of the other related disorders. So the fact that diagnoses are stable (meaning we're getting it "right" in the beginning) is encouraging for optimizing treatment planning.

Another factor that complicates diagnosis in schizophrenia is the considerable heterogeneity in presentation. There is considerable variability in how two different individuals diagnosed with schizophrenia will experience the disorder and in how a single individual will experience the disorder over their lifetime. This is another reason why it's more helpful to think about schizophrenia as a spectrum of experiences rather than a discrete condition.

Chapter 5

Relationship to Other Psychotic Disorders

Because schizophrenia exists on a spectrum, it is necessarily intertwined with related conditions. Although there are some nuances, the following are the major distinctions between schizophrenia and conditions often confused with it, all according to the DSM-5.

Schizoaffective Disorder, Major Depressive Disorder, and Bipolar Disorder with Psychotic Features

The distinction between schizophrenia, schizoaffective disorder, major depressive disorder with psychotic features, and bipolar disorder with psychotic features rests primarily on the severity, proportion, and timing of mood symptoms. Mood symptoms are things like depression or mania (mania is an *extremely* elevated mood usually associated with bipolar disorder).

Making an accurate distinction between schizophrenia and schizoaffective disorder isn't especially important because the clinical course of these conditions and the treatment approaches are very similar. But distinguishing between schizophrenia and mood disorders with psychotic features (i.e., major depressive disorder and bipolar disorder with psychotic features) is important because these conditions usually require a different treatment approach.

To be diagnosed with schizoaffective disorder, the person must have either a major depressive episode or a manic episode *at the same time* that they have symptoms of schizophrenia – delusions, hallucinations, disorganized speech or behavior, or negative symptoms. Plus, those symptoms of depression or mania must be present the *majority of the time* the person has the symptoms of schizophrenia. If the person doesn't have depression or mania that goes along with the psychotic symptoms or the depression/mania is present for only a brief period, they might have schizophrenia rather than schizoaffective disorder. Schizoaffective disorder also doesn't require that the person has a major decline in how they function at work, in their relationships, or in taking care of themselves, whereas schizophrenia does.

It is common for people with schizophrenia to have occasional symptoms of depression or mania. If the person *only* experiences psychotic symptoms (delusions, hallucinations, disorganized speech or behavior, or negative symptoms) when they're in the middle of a major depressive episode or a manic episode, the proper diagnosis might be major depressive disorder with psychotic features or bipolar disorder with psychotic features.

Unfortunately, many professionals think that if a person has psychotic symptoms and mood symptoms at the same time, that's sufficient to diagnose schizoaffective disorder, but that's not true. Both schizoaffective disorder and mood disorders with psychotic features (i.e., major depressive disorder with psychotic features and bipolar disorder with psychotic features) have that overlap when a person is experiencing mood symptoms and psychotic symptoms at the same time. **The difference is that with mood disorders with psychotic features, the psychotic features will *always* overlap with the mood symptoms.** In other words, they'll *only* ever experience hallucinations or delusions when they're also depressed or manic. If there are periods when the person has psychotic symptoms but *doesn't* have mood symptoms, then we're more likely dealing with schizophrenia or schizoaffective disorder.

One way to conceptualize the distinctions between schizophrenia, schizoaffective disorder, major depressive disorder with psychotic features, and bipolar disorder with psychotic features is like this:

PSYCHOTIC SYMPTOMS
↑

Schizophrenia
Mostly psychotic symptoms, without mania/depression symptoms

Schizoaffective Disorder
Psychotic symptoms with AND without depression/mania

Major Depressive Disorder or Bipolar Disorder with Psychotic Features
Mostly depression/mania symptoms, with psychotic symptoms ONLY during depression/mania

Major Depressive Disorder or Bipolar Disorder
Mostly depression/mania symptoms, without psychotic symptoms

↓
DEPRESSION/MANIA SYMPTOMS

During the first psychotic episode, it is often very difficult to make this diagnostic distinction because mood symptoms and agitation are very common in acute episodes of schizophrenia, and they're typical of schizoaffective disorder and mood disorders with psychotic features.

Schizophreniform Disorder and Brief Psychotic Disorder

The distinction between schizophrenia, schizophreniform disorder, and brief psychotic disorder rests primarily on the length of time symptoms have been present. A person must have had continuous *signs* of schizophrenia for at least *six* months, with *symptoms* present for a significant portion of time for *one* month to meet criteria for schizophrenia (*signs* are less severe and more general than *symptoms*). Schizophreniform disorder also requires that symptoms be present for a significant portion of time for one month but requires signs for *less than 6 months*. And brief psychotic disorder requires symptoms for at least one day but less than one month, with the person eventually returning to the same level of functioning they had prior to experiencing the symptoms. Here's what it looks like side-by-side.

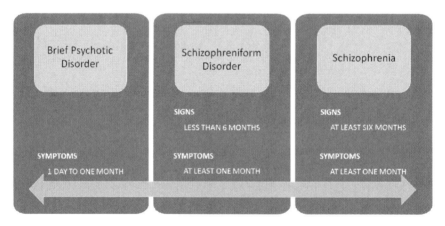

Delusional Disorder

People with delusional disorder have delusions, as you'd expect from the name. But it's very different than what's seen in schizophrenia. For one, the delusions in delusional disorder don't usually have the bizarre quality of the delusions in schizophrenia. Examples of bizarre delusions are that aliens have removed your brain or that satellites are inserting thoughts into your brain; these delusions are completely implausible. Examples of non-bizarre delusions are that the police are surveilling your house or a celebrity is infatuated with you; while *possible*, these delusions are highly improbable and don't have any evidence to support them. Also, whereas schizophrenia requires a person has at least *two* psychotic symptoms (delusions, hallucinations, disorganized speech, disorganized behavior, or negative symptoms), delusional disorder requires that the person has *only* had delusions. Plus, functioning is not impaired and behavior is not obviously bizarre in delusional disorder. Interestingly, while we saw earlier that schizophrenia is more common in men than women (14 men for every 10 women), delusional disorder is three times more common in women than men (10 men for every 30 women; reviewed in Combs & Mueser, 2007). Also, delusional disorder has an average age of onset 20 years later than schizophrenia (reviewed in Combs & Mueser, 2007).

Schizotypal Personality Disorder

In schizotypal personality disorder, the symptoms are typically subthreshold, meaning they aren't quite of the severity that's usually seen in schizophrenia. Plus, in schizotypal personality, the symptoms are usually associated with persistent personality features, whereas in schizophrenia the symptoms usually show up episodically. In other words, schizophrenia has *periods* of persistent psychotic symptoms, whereas in schizotypal personality disorder, the related behaviors are more pervasive.

Substance-Induced Psychotic Disorder

Substance use refers to introducing any sort of substance into the body, including alcohol, nicotine, caffeine, marijuana, prescription pills, inhalants, illicit substances, over-the-counter medications, etc. Certain substances can cause psychotic symptoms, either while the person is intoxicated from the substance or while they're withdrawing from the substance.

The distinction between schizophrenia and a substance-induced psychotic disorder is typically made by analyzing whether the psychotic symptoms start when the substance use starts, plus looking at whether the symptoms go away when the substance is withdrawn. This can be a really hard diagnostic distinction to make because people don't always have accurate information about their own substance use and they aren't always honest about their substance use. Plus, people with schizophrenia who use substances often have few or no periods of their life in which they *aren't* using substances, so there might not be a reliable period in their history to determine whether they continue to have symptoms of schizophrenia even when they aren't using substances (reviewed in Combs & Mueser, 2007). That can make it really difficult to confirm that they actually have schizophrenia rather than a substance use disorder.

Substances associated with psychotic disorders during intoxication include alcohol, cannabis, PCP and other hallucinogens, inhalants, sedatives/ hypnotics/ anxiolytics, and stimulants (including cocaine and amphetamine-type substances).

Substances associated with psychotic disorders during withdrawal include alcohol and sedatives/hypnotics/anxiolytics.

Chapter 6

Co-Occurring Conditions

From the above discussion, it's clear that schizophrenia can occur side-by-side with mood problems and substance use problems. Above, we were talking about how to determine whether a person has schizophrenia *or* another condition, but now it's time to talk about when a person has schizophrenia *and* another condition. When a person has two mental health conditions at once, we call that "comorbid" or "co-occurring" conditions.

When schizophrenia co-occurs with other mental health conditions, it's associated with increases in suicidal behavior and substance use (Kelleher et al., 2017). Between 20% and 50% of individuals with schizophrenia *attempt* suicide, and one out of every ten *dies* by suicide (reviewed in Lambert & Kinsley, 2011; and Silverstein et al., 2006). This is another reason why effective treatment of the entire schizophrenia condition (i.e., not just the symptoms, but the person as a whole, including their functional deficits and comorbid conditions) is so important. Risk for suicide is highest when the person with schizophrenia also has depression or mania, uses substances, has attempted suicide previously, is experiencing their first psychotic episode, or is just about to go into or be released from the hospital (reviewed in Combs & Mueser, 2007).

Depression

Schizophrenia frequently co-occurs with major depression, with between 25% and 33% of individuals with schizophrenia also meeting criteria for major depressive disorder in their lifetime (reviewed in Silverstein et al., 2006). In fact, depression so commonly co-occurs with schizophrenia that some models of schizophrenia actually have categories for symptoms of depression and mania (Shevlin et al., 2016) in addition to categories for positive, negative, and disorganized symptoms.

Depression can show up at any point in the illness -- from way before symptoms of schizophrenia ever show up to when the symptoms of schizophrenia are in remission -- but depression tends to get better as the symptoms of schizophrenia improve (reviewed in Combs & Mueser, 2007). Both conditions typically have onset in late adolescence and adulthood and both appear to have a similar genetic cause (Nivard et al., 2017).

As far as symptoms go, we see the strongest correlations between depression and paranoia, hallucinations, and disorganized thinking, with all these symptoms apparently sharing a genetic overlap (Zavos et al., 2016). And then we also see smaller correlations between depression and anhedonia (i.e., nothing feels fun or interesting) and other negative symptoms.

People with depression on top of schizophrenia tend to get admitted to the hospital more, are less likely to be employed, and experience more suicidality (reviewed in Combs & Mueser, 2007).

Anxiety

About 45% of individuals with schizophrenia also have anxiety (reviewed in Combs & Mueser, 2007), which can be an independent condition or can be secondary to the symptoms themselves. In other words, a person with schizophrenia might have anxiety that has nothing to do with the schizophrenia symptoms. Or they might have anxiety *about* their symptoms. For example, auditory hallucinations are often really frightening -- both the experience itself and the content of the hallucinations. That alone can create anxiety. But when auditory hallucinations command individuals to perform actions they would ordinarily consider immoral, anxiety is massive. Anxiety can also stem from the stress associated with prior psychotic episodes, which can be traumatic. And it's really common for people with schizophrenia to have social anxiety secondary to their deficits in social functioning. Further, anxiety might actually contribute to developing persecutory delusions (i.e., believing people are trying to hurt you) and hallucinations (reviewed in Combs & Mueser, 2007). Finally, approximately

15% to 25% of individuals with schizophrenia have obsessive-compulsive symptoms, and this usually is associated with poor response to treatment and poor functional outcomes (reviewed in Silverstein et al., 2006).

Substance Abuse

Substance use disorders are the most common co-occurring disorder for people with schizophrenia (Combs & Mueser, 2007). People with schizophrenia are four times more likely to have a substance use disorder than people in the general population (reviewed in Combs & Mueser, 2007). About half of the people with schizophrenia will have a substance use disorder in their lifetime, which can exacerbate the symptoms of schizophrenia and provoke a relapse of an acute episode of schizophrenia (reviewed in Combs & Mueser, 2007). Plus, having a substance use disorder along with schizophrenia means people go to the hospital more frequently, have more problems with housing and homelessness, are more vulnerable to violence, have more financial difficulties, and have more problems sticking to their treatment plans (reviewed in Combs & Mueser, 2007). But, compared to other people with substance use disorders, people with schizophrenia who use substances tend to use smaller quantities of drugs and alcohol and rarely develop physical dependence on the substances (reviewed in Combs & Mueser, 2007).

Approximately 80% to 90% of individuals with schizophrenia are reported to smoke cigarettes (reviewed in Lambert & Kinsley, 2011; reviewed in Silverstein et al., 2006). In part, this seems to be a way to reduce medication side effects and to correct some of the specific deficits associated with schizophrenia. For example, nicotine use lowers how much antipsychotic medications are in your blood, which then reduces side effects. Nicotine also improves cognitive functioning by stimulating certain neurotransmitter receptors in the brain that have been shown to be dysfunctional in individuals with schizophrenia (reviewed in Silverstein et al., 2006). Further, nicotine corrects sensory-gating deficits (reviewed in Lambert & Kinsley, 2011). It's a complicated process, but basically sensory-gating deficits are a dysfunction in your brain's ability to manage the startle response to stimuli that are somewhat expected. Here's how it works. When you go to the eye doctor and they puff that air on your eyeball, the first one is startling; the second one is a little bit less startling because of the sensory-gating deficit -- your brain reduces the startle response because it expects the stimulus. Sensory-gating deficits are common in schizophrenia, which makes it difficult for the brain to filter out irrelevant information (including things you hear, memories, and inner monologue). Nicotine corrects this, which is one reason people with schizophrenia might be drawn to smoke cigarettes.

Polydipsia

An unusual but somewhat common co-occurring condition in schizophrenia is polydipsia, which is a compulsion to drink water even though your body isn't actually thirsty. People with polydipsia are moved to drink water to the point they will drink from unsafe locations (e.g., toilet bowls). Up to 25% of individuals with schizophrenia have polydipsia (reviewed in Silverstein et al., 2006). This can cause sodium levels in the body to reduce to a dangerous level. Sodium is important for managing the volume of blood in the body, keeping the appropriate amount of water in your cells (not too much or too little), and helping nerves and muscles function. When sodium levels are too low, symptoms such as nausea, vomiting, seizures, and delirium can occur, and this can be fatal (Bhatia, Goyal, Saha, & Doval, 2017).

Physical Health Problems

Individuals with schizophrenia experience major physical health problems, some of which are secondary to substance use (e.g., the typical physical health problems that come from consistent cigarette use or excessive alcohol use), some of which are secondary to medication side effects (e.g., increased risk for diabetes and obesity; more on this in Chapter 17), and some of which seem to be related to the typical lifestyle of a person with schizophrenia. For example, poverty, inadequate attention to health, inadequate healthcare services, reduced access to healthcare, and malnutrition are all environmental factors that can negatively impact the person's physical health. Together, these physical health problems result in people with schizophrenia dying from natural causes (i.e., eliminating vehicle accidents or other accidents) at 1.5 times the expected rate (reviewed in Silverstein et al., 2006). They are especially likely to die from cardiovascular events (e.g., strokes or heart attacks; Vermeulen et al., 2018).

Chapter 7

Violence

Many people with schizophrenia are housed in jails, especially those who do not have family support and who have fallen through the cracks of public mental health services (reviewed in Combs & Mueser, 2007). There is a public perception that individuals with schizophrenia are prone to violence. In truth, there *is* a connection, and major behavior problems in childhood (e.g., things like unusually aggressive fighting, conning others, or forcing others into sexual activity) can predict that a person might develop schizophrenia later (reviewed in Combs & Mueser, 2007).

But the relationship between schizophrenia and violence is complicated. While there is an association between psychosis and violence, random assaults are really uncommon, and the targets of the violence are almost always family members (reviewed in Combs & Mueser, 2007). About 8% of people with schizophrenia engage in violence within the first 20 weeks following discharge from the hospital (the time when rates of violence are highest), and 14% engage in violence within the first year after discharge (reviewed in Combs & Mueser, 2007). But these rates are actually *lower* than for people with depression or bipolar disorder, and the vast majority of people with schizophrenia are not violent.

The relationship between psychosis and violence is explained by paranoia (Coid, Ullrich, Bebbington, Fazel, & Keers, 2016), **substance use, and treatment nonadherence** (reviewed in Combs & Mueser, 2007). That is, people who experience paranoia are more likely to be violent, whereas individuals who don't experience that symptom are not. Moreover, with effective treatment, this association diminishes.

People with schizophrenia are far more likely to be the *victims* of violence and violent crime than to be the perpetrators. Between 43% and 81% of individuals with schizophrenia report being victimized at some point in their lives (reviewed in Combs

& Mueser, 2007), including being the victims of child maltreatment (which we'll chat about more in Chapter 10, when we talk about risk factors for schizophrenia). Estimates of posttraumatic stress disorder among people with schizophrenia usually range from 29% to 43%. Women with schizophrenia and other severe mental illnesses are at especially high risk for being victimized, with as many as 77% to 97% of women who are sometimes homeless reporting they've been victimized (reviewed in Combs & Mueser, 2007).

Chapter 8

Insight

It is common for people with schizophrenia, especially during the times when symptoms are most severe, to lack insight into the nature of their symptoms and condition. This means they might not even be aware they have symptoms of schizophrenia; it's actually a lot like in dementia when a person doesn't know they are confused and have dementia.

According to at least one model (Lysaker et al., 2018), evidence suggests poor insight comes from problems integrating various sources of information. Specifically, if it's hard for you to make sense of information coming into your brain from the outside world, then it's hard to create a coherent understanding of yourself and others, which then interferes with how aware you are that you have a psychiatric condition. People with poor insight into their condition tend to abandon their treatment plans, which means they relapse more often, get committed to the hospital more often, show more aggression, have worse social functioning, and in general just fare worse.

People with poor insight into their condition often fail to stick to their treatment plans. But this isn't the only reason people have trouble following their treatment plans. The paranoia and distrust that can be a symptom of schizophrenia can make people with schizophrenia believe their doctors are dangerous or their medications are poisonous (reviewed in Combs & Mueser, 2007).

PART II

Causes, Risk Factors, & Pathophysiology

There are several theories about what causes schizophrenia, all with varying degrees of research support, and most suggesting that it's ultimately a brain disorder with malformations in both how the brain is *structured* and how it *functions* (Lambert & Kinsley, 2011). Currently, the field has massive datasets that are enhancing our knowledge about schizophrenia, including what causes it and what pathological physical processes keep it going. But even though these large datasets provide a wealth of information, they also complicate statistical analyses, so researchers are now making efforts to be mindful of the best ways to analyze this data and gather the most accurate conclusions (Krystal et al., 2017). The exact cause of schizophrenia remains unknown, but the following summarizes the current knowledge of what causes schizophrenia.

Chapter 9

Early Explanations

A neurodevelopmental approach to schizophrenia was developed in 1891 by Clouston (reviewed in Murray et al., 2017) but was quickly replaced by Kraepelin's conceptualization, which is typically considered the "first" explanation of schizophrenia. This is ironic because now that earlier neurodevelopmental approach is one of the leading conceptualizations of schizophrenia (more on that later).

Schizophrenia was initially called "dementia praecox" by Kraepelin (1893), who thought of schizophrenia as an early form of dementia. He thought that schizophrenia was a degenerative process that got worse and worse over a person's life. We pretty quickly figured out that wasn't true. [Side note: We're just now learning that there is some specific degeneration in the brain over the course of schizophrenia. However, that seems to be caused by antipsychotic medications, substance use, and unhealthy lifestyle choices of people living with schizophrenia, not to effects of schizophrenia itself (reviewed in Murray et al., 2017).]

So once it was clear schizophrenia was not a degenerative process like dementia, it was reconceptualized. Bleuler (1911), noticing the differences in how the symptoms show up across different people and across one person's lifespan, conceptualized schizophrenia as a family of related disorders, much like our current understanding of the condition (see Chapter 4). He then renamed the condition "schizophrenia," which translates to "split mind." This has led to the unfortunate association between schizophrenia and dissociative identity or multiple personality, which is a completely different experience. **What Bleuler meant by "split mind" was that the person's emotional and cognitive processes were not operating in a logical or synchronized fashion, which causes the cluster of illogical symptoms of schizophrenia.** This hypothesis actually coordinates well with current hypotheses about asynchrony and poor communication among various brain processes.

Chapter 10

Risk Factors

Predicting which people will ultimately develop schizophrenia starts with examining risk factors. Obviously, the more risk factors for schizophrenia a person has, the greater their odds of having psychotic experiences (Pries et al., 2018). Negative symptoms and emotion dysregulation (e.g., moodiness, difficulty regulating anger or sadness) increase how much the following risk factors affect psychotic experiences (Pries et al., 2018).

Genetic Risk Factors

There has been considerable interest and effort in understanding the genetic underpinnings of schizophrenia. With schizophrenia existing on a continuum with normal experience, evidence has shown that genetic susceptibility to schizophrenia and related disorders can be found even in individuals who don't meet diagnostic criteria (Ortega-Alonso et al., 2017). In the next three chapters, we'll discuss some of the brain abnormalities that occur in schizophrenia, but in examining the genetics of schizophrenia, it's important to note that the genes responsible for schizophrenia change the way the brain *works*. Specifically, in all human brains, the neurons change and build new connections throughout life to adjust to new situations or to compensate for damage, injury, or disease. We call that process *neuroplasticity*. There is a theory (reviewed in Silverstein et al., 2006) that the brain of a person with schizophrenia is even *more* plastic than most, meaning it is changing even more than the average person's brain. This could then mean that the brain of a person with schizophrenia is even more reactive to stress than the average person's brain. Keep this in mind as you review the following genetic evidence because the genes don't just code for whether a person "has" or "doesn't have" schizophrenia; they code for how the brain works, including how it responds to stress.

Family Studies

Although about 1% of the world's population has schizophrenia, the diagnosis tends to cluster in families (reviewed in Lambert & Kinsley, 2011). In fact, while most people have a 1% chance of developing schizophrenia, if your parent has schizophrenia, your risk increases to 10% (reviewed in Silverstein et al., 2006).

Twin studies

Examinations of twins are useful for understanding genetic underpinnings. Identical twins (called monozygotic) have 100% the same DNA, so any differences between the twins can be attributed to the environment (e.g., how and where they grew up, what they've eaten in their lives, how they've taken care of themselves, illnesses they've contracted, etc.) rather than genes.

If there is a 100% concordance rate, this means that 100% of the time a given characteristic will be shared between identical twins; if there is a 0% concordance rate, this means that the twins will *never* share the same characteristic. In reality, concordance rates are almost never 0% or 100%. In schizophrenia, the concordance rate is 48%, meaning *if a twin is diagnosed with schizophrenia, there is a 48% chance their twin will also be diagnosed with schizophrenia*. Let's talk about why this figure is 48% rather than 100%. One reason that twins won't always be diagnosed in pairs is that although identical twins' *genes* are identical, the way their body *expresses* those genes is imprecise and may not be identical. It's similar to how one film director interprets a screenplay differently than another; same screenplay, different movie. Also, the diagnostic criteria themselves are imprecise and open to interpretation, which can create diagnostic uncertainty. And two individuals can express symptoms differently, with one resulting in a diagnosis of schizophrenia and the other not. Finally, twins, even when raised in the same household, can have different birth complications, medical histories, and life experiences that affect risk for schizophrenia.

The idea that schizophrenia is caused by one gene was relatively quickly dismissed in favor of the reality that schizophrenia is mediated by *numerous* genetic variants, most with a very small effect and perhaps a few having a larger effect (reviewed in Murray et al., 2017). Currently, there appear to be genetic links on several chromosomes, including 1, 6, 8, 10, 13, 15, 18, 22, and X, some of which control neurotransmitter transmission or regulate proteins involved in neuron synapses (Lambert & Kinsley, 2011). Lots of complicated words in that sentence, but basically some of the genes control how the brain works and how it sends messages across the brain and body.

Genetic markers are genes that are associated with some sort of observable variation. So we have genetic markers for eye color and breast cancer and height and just about every other trait and behavior. The genetic markers for schizophrenia overlap with genetic markers for related psychiatric conditions, such as bipolar disorder and autism (Lambert & Kinsley, 2011). This means it's likely that there are several general genes that cause nonspecific changes throughout the brain and body, and when these changes accumulate they sometimes cause schizophrenia. We also know that changes in intellectual ability and brain structure and function are important genetic markers for risk for schizophrenia (reviewed in Bohlken, Brouwer, Mandl, Kahn, & Pol, 2016).

Ventricles are cavities in the brain filled with cerebrospinal fluid; they're sort of like swimming pools in the brain. We've known for a long time that identical twins with schizophrenia have larger cerebral ventricles than their twins without schizophrenia, which suggests the ventricle enlargement isn't caused by genes (because they have 100% the same genes) but instead is caused by something in the environment (reviewed in Murray et al., 2017). This hypothesis was further supported by evidence that the twins with schizophrenia tend to have been exposed to more severe problems in the weeks around birth. Those kind of adverse life experiences can change how the brain then develops. In other words, the twin's brain starts reading that screenplay differently than the other twin's brain does.

A defect on chromosome 22 has garnered particular investigation. 22q11.2 deletion syndrome (also known as DiGeorge syndrome and velocardiofacial syndrome) is a disorder caused by the deletion of a small portion of chromosome 22. Nearly one-third of individuals with this syndrome develop a psychotic disorder in their lifetime (Murray et al., 2017; Weisman et al., 2017), and many of them develop schizophrenia.

Environmental Risk Factors

If schizophrenia were caused exclusively by genetic factors, identical twins would always be diagnosed in pairs. In reality, schizophrenia is caused by a combination of genetic factors and environmental risk factors. In fact, animals begin showing schizophrenia symptoms when they have genetic abnormalities that cause dopamine dysfunction *and* they're exposed to moderate stress (Tan et al., 2018). This is because environmental factors (like stress) can actually alter how the brain develops, how it functions, and how the genes are expressed, particularly in the brain areas implicated in schizophrenia, like the hippocampus (reviewed in Silverstein et al., 2006).

Developmental Trauma

Exposure to severe stress has immediate and enduring negative effects on learning, behavior, and health. The relationship between stress and psychosis is especially strong for childhood trauma (reviewed in Bailey et al., 2018), and people with schizophrenia are known to have high rates of neglect and physical and sexual abuse in childhood (reviewed in Silverstein et al., 2006). People with schizophrenia who endured especially severe abuse were more likely to have poor functioning even before they ever developed schizophrenia and are more likely to have cognitive deficits (reviewed in Silverstein et al., 2006). People who have schizophrenia that were traumatized in childhood tend to have more severe hallucinations and delusions, but childhood trauma isn't associated with negative symptoms (Bailey et al., 2018). Instead, children who were *neglected* in childhood were more likely to have negative symptoms of psychosis (Bailey et al., 2018). There is a specific link between childhood *sexual* abuse and *auditory* hallucinations and between childhood *emotional* abuse and *delusions* (Hardy et al., 2016). Interestingly, that study didn't find any associations between childhood *physical* abuse and psychotic symptoms. Loss of a parent, bullying, and social exclusion are other adverse childhood experiences that can increase risk for schizophrenia (Selten, Booij, Buwalda, & Meyer-Lindenberg, 2017; and reviewed in Murray et al., 2017).

The research evidence generally suggests this relationship between schizophrenia and trauma is more than just an association or correlation. In fact, it seems trauma (especially childhood trauma) can actually *cause* psychosis (Gibson, Alloy, & Ellman, 2016; Hardy et al., 2016), though more evidence is needed to confirm this. This could be because people with schizophrenia are more sensitive to stress (Veling, Pot-Kolder, Counotte, Os, & Gaag, 2016; also reviewed in Murray et al., 2017). Alternatively, stress caused by abuse damages the hippocampus, which is a part of the brain important in long-term memories. This damage can cause memories of abuse experiences to lose some specific details that make them recognizable as memories, and that process can result in hallucinations (reviewed in Silverstein et al., 2006). Another proposed pathway from trauma to psychosis is through more general psychopathology, especially anxiety. For example, childhood trauma connects to symptoms such as grandiosity, excitement, and hostility via poor impulse control; and childhood neglect connects to negative symptoms via motor slowness (Isvoranu, Borkulo, et al., 2016). Most likely, however, exposure to trauma leads to psychosis through many pathways that intersect with other risk factors (environmental, genetic, etc.; Gibson et al., 2016).

It's worth noting that there are gender differences in victimization. Women are far more likely to be abused than men, especially with respect to sexual abuse/assault and domestic violence (reviewed in Combs & Mueser, 2007). They are also more likely to become dependent on the perpetrators of their abuse (e.g., being financially dependent on an abusive paramour), which can result in chronic victimization. Plus, people who are abuse victims often don't report their abuse to treatment providers or even friends and family, so it can be difficult to determine whether this plays a role in the development or exacerbation of their psychotic symptoms.

Related to developmental trauma is the concept of "high expressed emotion" in families. We usually think of expressing emotions as a good thing, but expressed emotion in this context refers to family members that are hostile, critical, or emotionally overinvolved. This type of family context has consistently been shown to be an important stressor increasing the risk for relapse and rehospitalization in schizophrenia (Ng, Yeung, & Gao, 2019).

Living Environment

There has been a consistent finding that being born in an urban area, growing up in an urban area, and moving to an urban area increase risk for schizophrenia (reviewed in Silverstein et al., 2006). In fact, being raised in an urban area *doubles* risk for schizophrenia as an adult compared to being raised in rural areas (Newbury et al., 2016; Newbury et al., 2017). Further, it seems the *degree* of urbanicity affects risk for psychosis (i.e., the more "urban" the area, the greater the risk; reviewed in Murray et al., 2017). And this is not because of substance use in urban areas or because urban areas have larger populations of people with mental illness (reviewed in Silverstein et al., 2006). Rather, this appears to result from a combination of the social conditions of living in urban areas (e.g., poverty, higher crime rates, low sense of community or social cohesion, social isolation) plus the increased likelihood of being the victim of a violent crime (Newbury et al., 2016; Newbury et al., 2017), which can create the stress that ultimately kickstarts the schizophrenia process.

Just as migrating to an urban area increases risk for schizophrenia, moving to a new country can increase risk for schizophrenia (reviewed in Silverstein et al., 2006). This is especially true for people moving from *developing* countries to *developed* countries. More than 90% of people with schizophrenia are living in developing (as opposed to developed) countries (Lambert & Kinsley, 2011), but people with schizophrenia in developed countries tend to have greater levels of disability associated with the condition (reviewed in Silverstein et al., 2006). In other words, people in developing countries with schizophrenia actually have a better prognosis and course of illness (reviewed in Combs & Mueser, 2007). We don't know exactly why this is, but current theories (reviewed in Combs & Mueser, 2007) suggest it could be because stigma and social rejection associated with having a severe mental illness vary across cultures, there are differences in family and community (e.g., neighborhood, religious) support across cultures, and certain cultures are much more accepting of psychotic phenomena, which reduces the burden of experiencing those symptoms.

Being an underprivileged minority also is associated with increased risk for schizophrenia (reviewed in Silverstein et al., 2006). This is thought to be true because these individuals experience more social defeat and long-term stress, which increases dopamine in the areas of the brain that are important in schizophrenia physiology (more on that in Chapter 12).

Cannabis Use

The most specific paths we know between environmental risk factors and symptoms of schizophrenia involve cannabis use (Isvoranu, Borsboom, Os, & Guloksuz, 2016). Importantly, cannabis doesn't just produce psychotic symptoms during intoxication or withdrawal; it has been shown to induce *chronic* psychotic disorders (Marconi, Forti, Lewis, Murray, & Vassos, 2016). **In *every single study* in a recent meta-analysis, cannabis was shown to be associated with increased risk for psychosis** (Marconi et al., 2016). In fact, cannabis use (especially high-potency and synthetic varieties) *doubles* the risk for schizophrenia by interacting with a specific gene (reviewed in Silverstein et al., 2006). Moreover, the risk increases in a dose-response fashion (Marconi et al., 2016; also reviewed in Murray et al., 2017), meaning the more cannabis a person uses, the higher the risk for schizophrenia. It has been estimated that if no one smoked marijuana, 8% to 25% of cases of schizophrenia could be prevented altogether (reviewed in Murray et al., 2017), highlighting the importance of education about cannabis use, particularly in the current climate aimed at decriminalizing and legalizing marijuana use.

Chapter 11

Neuroanatomy

Now that we know some of the factors that increase risk for schizophrenia, including some of the genetic factors that create differences in the schizophrenia brain, it's time to move on to talking more specifically about what the schizophrenia brain looks like.

Individuals with schizophrenia have significant differences in how their brains are structured, but we don't know exactly what causes these differences. Let's start with the cortex. The cortex is the outer part of the brain with all the wrinkles that has the four primary lobes of the brain: the frontal, parietal, occipital, and temporal lobes. **Individuals with schizophrenia tend to have less volume in the brain's cortex.** In fact, this represents atrophy, which means the cortex actually got *smaller* over time (as opposed to just never developed to a normal size). This loss in cortical volume occurs in late adolescence and early adulthood during the onset of schizophrenia (Murray et al., 2017). Plus, volume reductions specifically in the frontal lobe (that's the part behind your forehead) are associated with apathy, inattention, motor deficiencies, lack of spontaneity, and reduction in general motivation (reviewed in Lambert & Kinsley, 2011) -- in short, negative symptoms. And people with schizophrenia who have abnormalities in their gyri (those are the valleys between the wrinkles on the surface of the brain) tend to have a poorer response to treatment (Murray et al., 2017). Interestingly, when the volume reductions extend from the cortex to the subcortex (that's the part of the brain below the wrinkles, where you find the limbic system, hypothalamus, and lots of other structures), those people tend to have longer illnesses and more negative symptoms compared to people who only have volume reductions in the cortex (Dwyer et al., 2018).

Another anatomical marker of schizophrenia is enlarged ventricles. As we talked about in Chapter 10, ventricles are cavities in the brain filled with cerebrospinal fluid that are part of the brain's circulatory system and are involved in protecting the brain from injuries. When these ventricles are enlarged, they operate as a balloon and compress the surrounding tissue, which can eventually cause that tissue to atrophy (reviewed in Lambert & Kinsley, 2011; reviewed in Rosenzweig, Breedlove, & Watson, 2005). Research shows in at least some cases ventricular enlargement is caused by brain bleeding in newborns who are born prematurely or experience low levels of oxygen in their blood (reviewed in Murray et al., 2017).

The cerebellum is a structure on the back of the brain that looks like another tiny brain tucked under the cortex. It's involved in regulating motor movement. **In schizophrenia, the mid-portion of the cerebellum is smaller** (reviewed in Lambert & Kinsley, 2011), which could explain some of the motor symptoms of schizophrenia (see Chapter 1).

As we all know, stress increases cortisol, the "stress hormone" that is implicated in heart disease. Further, chronically increased cortisol can damage the hippocampus, which is involved in making long-term memories and has been implicated in a variety of schizophrenia symptoms. Most notably, if the hippocampus is damaged, memories may lose their contextual information and, when memories are activated, can be experienced as hallucinations (reviewed in Silverstein et al., 2006). Further, a damaged hippocampus can change how the self is experienced. Not only do people with schizophrenia have a smaller hippocampus, but they also have a smaller amygdala, which is involved in detecting fear and preparing for emergencies (reviewed in Rosenzweig et al., 2005).

Chapter 12

Neurophysiology

It's not just the structure of the brain that's amiss in schizophrenia, it's also how it *functions*. And just as there are lots of genetic markers for schizophrenia, schizophrenia is not isolated to problems in a specific brain structure. Instead, it is the result of problematic interactions *between* structures. Connectivity across the brain is disturbed in schizophrenia, leading to disruptions in functioning throughout the brain (Klauser et al., 2016). The areas most implicated include the frontal lobes, temporal lobes, basal ganglia, and possibly also the cerebellum, thalamus, and hippocampus (reviewed in Silverstein et al., 2006). When there are widespread abnormalities in how these areas coordinate with each other to transmit messages, symptoms of schizophrenia can present. Specifically, when neurons are disrupted (either because there are too few of them, they're disorganized, they're the wrong size, or they're not able to transmit messages clearly), the signals can become distorted as they move through the brain. As a result of this poor operation, hallucinations, distorted thinking, and paranoia occur (reviewed in Lambert & Kinsley, 2011). It's actually a lot like the childhood game of telephone -- if there's any disruption or lack of clarity in how messages are transmitted, the message that gets to the end of the line can be totally different than the one we started with.

As mentioned, the frontal lobe is one of the areas most implicated in schizophrenia pathology. The frontal lobe has a lot of responsibilities, including controlling other parts of the brain. You can think of it as the brain's switchboard or control panel. When the frontal lobe is less active than normal, negative symptoms can occur. And reductions in a specific part of the frontal lobe (the medial frontal gyrus) results in problems with setting, accomplishing, and re-evaluating goals (Poppe et al., 2016). Ordinarily, the prefrontal cortex inhibits activity in the limbic system. When it's not doing such a great job at this, hallucinations can occur (reviewed in Silverstein et al.,

2006). Among people experiencing their first episode of schizophrenia, about 90% of the brain dysfunction (in terms of how the brain operates with respect to physiology and connectivity) is in the frontal lobe, whereas for individuals with more chronic schizophrenia the dysfunction broadens (Li et al., 2016).

Evidence shows auditory hallucinations (e.g., hearing voices) are caused by excessive activity in the brain's temporal and auditory lobes, which are highly involved in auditory processing and various language processes, as well as in several other areas (the orbitofrontal cortex, cingulate cortex, and limbic and striatal structures; reviewed in Lambert & Kinsley, 2011).

The thalamus is involved in sending sensory information -- like sights and sounds -- to its appropriate destination in the brain, and it also regulates sleep and alertness. Changes in the thalamus aren't usually observed early in schizophrenia but become prominent in chronic schizophrenia (Li et al., 2016). *Reduced* connectivity between the thalamus and *frontal lobe* correlates with positive symptoms of schizophrenia; *increased* connectivity between the thalamus and *temporal lobe* correlates with negative symptoms of schizophrenia; and *increased* connectivity between the thalamus and *sensory-motor cortex* correlates with general symptoms of schizophrenia (Li et al., 2016).

Basic Neuroscience Review

We need to take a brief break to do some basic neuroscience review. The cells in the brain are called neurons. They have tiny gaps between each other, called synapses. When a neuron wants to send a message to another neuron, the first neuron packages up a chemical called a neurotransmitter. It pushes the neurotransmitter out into the synapse, and a receptor on the second neuron sucks it up. This process continues until the message reaches its destination. There are many types of neurotransmitters, but the important ones to know for schizophrenia are acetylcholine, norepinephrine, epinephrine, dopamine, serotonin, GABA, and glutamate. Neurons that use certain types of neurotransmitters are organized into "systems" (i.e., dopamine system, glutamatergic system).

Dopamine Hypothesis

The dopamine hypothesis of schizophrenia has been one of the most influential theories about what causes schizophrenia. **This hypothesis posited that schizophrenia symptoms were due to excessive levels of dopamine in the brain.** Like many medical theories, this theory developed by accident, when it was observed that thorazine, a medication used to calm anesthetized surgery patients, was also helpful in controlling psychotic symptoms and was known to work by keeping neurons from releasing or receiving dopamine. Ordinarily, when messages are transmitted from one neuron to the next, there is some extra neurotransmitter left in the gap between neurons that is recycled by the first neuron and used again later. The hypothesis developed that this extra dopamine was not being cleared adequately or quickly enough, which resulted in extra stimulation or firings of that next neuron (reviewed in Lambert & Kinsley, 2011). It's kind of like if no one takes the potato chips away from us, we just keep eating them. The dopamine hypothesis was further supported by observations that drugs that result in temporarily high levels of dopamine (like cocaine or methamphetamine) create psychotic symptoms during intoxication and by observations that increasing dopamine levels in the brain (e.g., by keeping that extra dopamine from being recycled or releasing extra dopamine into the synapse) create psychotic symptoms (reviewed in Lambert & Kinsley, 2011). And when individuals with Parkinson's disease are given too much of the medication L-dopa (which increases dopamine levels in the brain), psychotic symptoms can develop (reviewed in Silverstein et al., 2006). It is also known that certain areas of the brain (e.g., the associative striatum) create more dopamine than they should, an abnormality that can be seen at the very onset of prodromal symptoms and that increases as the first psychotic episode develops (reviewed in Murray et al., 2017). Finally, some genes implicated in schizophrenia affect dopamine directly, for example by affecting dopamine receptors or how dopamine signals are transmitted across the brain.

Despite there being evidence supporting the dopamine hypothesis, it ultimately didn't sufficiently explain the complexities of schizophrenia. For example, if excessive dopamine were the entire cause of schizophrenia, then blocking dopamine transmission should relieve the symptoms. While this improves symptoms, it doesn't alleviate them completely. Further, actually there is evidence of *reduced* dopamine in certain parts of the schizophrenia brain (reviewed in Lambert & Kinsley, 2011). More recent evidence suggests reduced dopamine levels in certain parts may lead to negative symptoms, while excessive dopamine levels in other parts may lead to positive symptoms (reviewed in Lambert & Kinsley, 2011). Finally, medications that are successful in treating schizophrenia symptoms don't target dopamine receptors exclusively, and several neurotransmitter systems (and interactions among them) are likely involved, including serotonin, glutamate, and acetylcholine.

Glutamate Dysfunction

With the dopamine hypothesis not receiving much support for explaining schizophrenia, attention turned toward glutamate and the NMDA receptor. NMDA receptors bind to glutamate and are involved in controlling memory and how synapses adjust to experience. When these receptors are underactive, there can be major changes in how neurons connect to each other and communicate (reviewed in Silverstein et al., 2006). This is because this type of receptor is involved in adapting to experience and making connections between cells. Also, several of the genes that are implicated in schizophrenia operate on the glutamatergic systems (Murray et al., 2017). It comes back around to dopamine, though, because the glutamatergic systems (i.e., the groups of neurons that communicate with glutamate) influence how dopamine is created and released.

Chapter 13

Neurodevelopment

One of the most influential theories of schizophrenia is that it is not just a dysfunction in how the brain is structured or how it functions but that schizophrenia represents an entire developmental process.

Evidence for its being a neurodevelopmental condition comes from observations that people who ultimately are diagnosed with schizophrenia have certain pregnancy and birth complications, such as bleeding, insufficient oxygen, low birth weight, reduced head size, and gestational stress (reviewed in Murray et al., 2017; and Silverstein et al., 2006). They also display minor indicators of neurological dysfunction, show problems with neuromotor development in early childhood, and have minor physical anomalies at birth (reviewed in Murray et al., 2017; and Silverstein et al., 2006). For example, individuals who eventually develop schizophrenia show more negative facial expressions during their first year of life and can be seen to have subtle abnormalities in muscle tone or muscle symmetry in their first two years of life (reviewed in Lambert & Kinsley, 2011). Oddly, they also have abnormalities in nail bed capillaries and fingerprints, which is thought to be a neurodevelopmental anomaly because fingerprints develop so early in gestation. Interestingly, they're also more likely to be ambidextrous and they show cognitive deficits (memory for verbal information, attention) by ages 7 to 12 (reviewed in Combs & Mueser, 2007). Not everyone shows these developmental markers for schizophrenia, and actually the early signs of schizophrenia are likely subtle, irregular, and gradual in onset and become more apparent as the onset of the acute phase of the illness looms (reviewed in Combs & Mueser, 2007).

Another piece of evidence for the neurodevelopmental hypothesis is that childhood mental health conditions tend to develop into more severe adult mental health conditions, such as schizophrenia, pointing to a common genetic origin and a developmental process (Nivard et al., 2017). And individuals at very high risk for developing schizophrenia show cognitive impairments that can predict later transition to schizophrenia (reviewed in Loewy et al., 2016), indicating the progression to schizophrenia begins long before the symptoms of the condition ever show up.

Many of the genes associated with schizophrenia affect brain development, especially cognitive development (reviewed in Murray et al., 2017). During development, brain cells grow, mature, and eventually migrate to their final destination in the brain. But in schizophrenia, the cells do not migrate correctly and do not arrive in the correct orientation (reviewed in Lambert & Kinsley, 2011), which means cells that ordinarily are highly organized look tangled and disorganized. This disorganization in structure creates monumental disorganization in information processing, with some messages being sent before they are ready, others being overprocessed, and some being changed altogether (reviewed in Lambert & Kinsley, 2011). Ultimately, this presents as the symptoms of schizophrenia.

In late adolescence, as brain development finalizes, our brains eliminate extra neurons and synaptic connections to increase the efficiency of message transmissions across the brain, a process called synaptic pruning. Adolescents who are normally developing lose approximately 1% of their brains' gray matter per year during this process (reviewed in Lambert & Kinsley, 2011). It has been proposed that schizophrenia results from problematic, possibly excessive, synaptic pruning, which may be caused by a variation in certain genes (human complement component C4) (reviewed in Murray et al., 2017). Further, the extent of this excessive pruning tends to be associated with the severity of a person's positive and negative symptoms (reviewed in Lambert & Kinsley, 2011).

Near the end of life, the positive symptoms of schizophrenia tend to lessen and problems with movement become more prominent, which suggests schizophrenia changes over the lifespan and the most prominent symptoms correspond to the part of the brain most metabolically active at that developmental stage (reviewed in Silverstein et al., 2006).

Further evidence for schizophrenia as a neurodevelopmental condition comes from confirmation that individuals with schizophrenia tend to have more birth complications (e.g., lower birth weight, oxygen deprivation), even among identical twins (i.e., the twin who develops schizophrenia had more birth complications than the twin who did not) (reviewed in Murray et al., 2017). Plus, environmental stress during gestation is correlated with developing schizophrenia (reviewed in Silverstein et al., 2006). This can include things like droughts and famines that affect maternal nutrition or even invasions or other war-related stress that affects general safety.

One implication of the neurodevelopmental theory is that by the time people are diagnosed and treated with medications, the illness has been progressing for an extended period, so the acute "onset" of the illness actually represents a later stage in the development of schizophrenia (Lambert & Kinsley, 2011).

Neural Diathesis-Stress Model of Schizophrenia

Diathesis-stress models of mental illness propose that mental illness results from a complex interaction between biological or genetic vulnerability (diathesis) and environmental or psychological factors (stress).

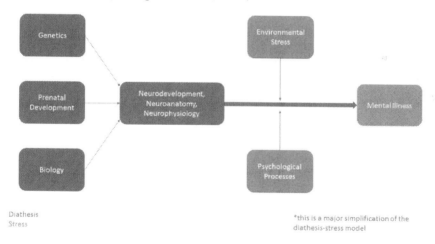

*this is a major simplification of the diathesis-stress model

The neural diathesis-stress model of schizophrenia (reviewed in Lambert & Kinsley, 2011) is an extension of this that emphasizes the role of *hormones* as the diathesis. Specifically, there are dramatic changes in steroidal hormones (testosterone, progesterone, estradiol, cortisol, and related hormones) at puberty, and adolescence is clearly known to be a critical phase in the development of schizophrenia. Basically, this model proposes that alterations in these hormones interfere with normal development. For example, some of these hormones increase dopamine synthesis or alter dopamine receptors in the brain, which can then create symptoms of schizophrenia (see Chapter 12). On the "stress" end, evidence shows that when we experience recurrent abuse or stress during development, our brains may become especially sensitive in responding to stress in adulthood, which can then result in schizophrenia symptoms.

Developmental Risk Factor Model of Schizophrenia

Most recently, the neurodevelopmental model of schizophrenia has transitioned into the *developmental risk factor model of schizophrenia* (reviewed in Murray et al., 2017). It works like this. Certain neurodevelopmental risk factors for schizophrenia (think: genes, early gestational age, birth complications, etc.) interact with environmental risk factors for schizophrenia (think: poverty, social stress, trauma, substance use) during development. These factors are present in childhood and affect how these children perform in school and how they interact with peers. Children who ultimately develop schizophrenia gradually fall increasingly behind their peers in their cognitive abilities. As they become differentiated (and isolated) from their peers, they often begin using substances, experience trauma, or have some other major adverse life experience. This affects the structure and function of their brains, including how their brains release dopamine and whether certain random experiences are misinterpreted as important. Plus, the events of their lives may make them interpret information in an unusual way, like becoming paranoid about random experiences. The stress associated with those initial symptoms further affects the structure and function of their brains, which causes more experiential misinterpretation, which causes more stress and creates a downward spiral into schizophrenia.

Chapter 14

Viral & Immunological Theory

Another classic theory of schizophrenia is the viral theory. **Mothers who are exposed to influenza, especially during the fifth month of pregnancy, are more likely to give birth to a child who eventually develops schizophrenia.** This hypothesis regarding exposure to a virus during a critical stage of fetal development is one theory of schizophrenia etiology (reviewed in Lambert & Kinsley, 2011).

There is also some evidence of retroviral activity in schizophrenia (reviewed in Silverstein et al., 2006). A retrovirus is a specific type of virus that becomes part of the person's genome and alters how genes are expressed.

So, these viral hypotheses propose that viral infection during a specific period in development might disrupt the very fragile process during which neurons are created and migrate to their ultimate destinations. It is thought this could occur because viruses operate by altering DNA, which could interfere with development in brain structure and function.

An extension of this idea that prenatal exposure to viruses leads to schizophrenia is evidence that schizophrenia (like many other mental health conditions) is associated with dysfunction in the immune system (reviewed in Wang & Miller, 2017). That is, abnormal immune responses to viral infection may change brain tissue and function and ultimately cause psychopathology (reviewed in Silverstein et al., 2006). Overall, however, there's very little evidence supporting these viral and immunological theories of schizophrenia (Silverstein et al., 2006).

PART III

Treatment

Chapter 15

Medical Model vs. Psychiatric Rehabilitation

Traditionally, treatment of schizophrenia has followed a "medical model," which treats schizophrenia as though it were a physical condition. The medical model has a few important assumptions (reviewed in Silverstein et al., 2006):

1. The *symptoms* of schizophrenia are the most important treatment targets
2. Medications are the primary (or even sole) treatment approach for schizophrenia
3. Treatment focuses on identifying and removing signs and symptoms of schizophrenia through medicine

This model neglects some important information about how schizophrenia develops, is experienced, and is expressed. An alternative model is "psychiatric rehabilitation," which treats schizophrenia as a much broader condition. Psychiatric rehabilitation has a few important assumptions (reviewed in Silverstein et al., 2006):

1. Real-world, community functioning is the most important treatment outcome
2. A variety of specific interventions are used to improve coping and behavior
3. Treatment focuses on reducing disability and promoting more effective functioning in the community

The concept of *recovery* is central to psychiatric rehabilitation. Traditionally, "recovery" from a condition has meant someone is "asymptomatic." For example, if you recover from a cold, it means you no longer have the sniffles. But over the past few decades, the word has come to have a much broader definition, with people living with schizophrenia feeling empowered to define recovery individually. To many, the definition continues to reflect a goal of symptom remission. To some, however, recovery means having a full-time job, even if some symptoms persist. To others, recovery means having fulfilling relationships. And to others, recovery means pursuing purposeful, meaningful activities. The concept here is much more focused on reducing the disability caused by the symptoms rather than eliminating the symptoms themselves. By this definition, between 21% and 57% of people with schizophrenia show periodic episodes of recovery whereby their symptoms are improved and they function better socially, educationally, and occupationally (reviewed in Combs & Mueser, 2007). And some of those even have extended periods of recovery without mental health treatment (reviewed in Combs & Mueser, 2007).

Conceptualized in this manner (reduced disability versus symptom remission), treatment approaches may be very different. An important component of the recovery model is that the individual with schizophrenia is a key member of the treatment team. This is because they make their personal definition of recovery and are instrumental in setting their recovery goals; the remaining treatment team members serve to suggest and implement strategies to reach those goals. When treatment plans are developed collaboratively, with the recovering individual, significant functional improvements can occur.

We can't really predict who is going to recover from schizophrenia or respond the best to treatment. This is because schizophrenia itself, as we've seen, is caused by so many factors interacting with each other, so recovering from schizophrenia involves addressing lots of interacting factors. But factors like sticking to a treatment plan, using alcohol or cigarettes or drugs, being exposed to a hostile or critical environment, and having psychosocial services available all affect how well a person will respond to treatment (reviewed in Combs & Mueser, 2007).

Chapter 16

Treatment Planning

Horrifically, fewer than 50% of individuals who are diagnosed with schizophrenia are receiving care or treatment (reported in Lambert & Kinsley, 2011). And of course schizophrenia tends to be associated with lifelong disability, especially among people who are not receiving intensive, evidence-based, recovery-oriented rehabilitation services (reviewed in Silverstein et al., 2006). So, improving outcomes is directly tied to the quality of the treatment plan and the services it assigns to the individual.

In the psychiatric rehabilitation model, treatment planning is intended to be a collaborative process between the person diagnosed with schizophrenia and other members of their treatment team. The process begins with articulating the person's recovery goals and then identifying their skills, interests, and treatment preferences. Then, we assess their deficits, impairments, disabilities, and other problems. Finally, we combine all that data and select treatment modalities that will rehabilitate the areas of need and move the person toward their recovery goals by using their strengths. Although it's extremely uncommon for treatment planning to resemble this described process, it is the most consistent with the recovery model and the most hypothesis-driven and data-driven strategy. Let's discuss this process in more detail.

Step 1: Identify Client's Phase of Illness

Ideally, treatment begins by identifying people who are at clinical high risk for developing a psychotic disorder (see Chapter 10). However, among those who are at very high risk, it remains very difficult to distinguish those who will eventually develop schizophrenia from those who will not, despite being at high risk. Nevertheless, it's important for treatment planning to adjust for the stage of the illness the individual is in. For example, individuals who are at clinical high risk for developing a psychotic disorder have different needs than individuals who are in the prodromal phase of the illness (e.g., when the illness is just budding), the acute phase of the illness (e.g., florid psychotic symptoms are present), the stabilizing or stable phase (e.g., symptoms are present but are responding to treatment), or the remission phase (e.g., symptoms have died down); and all of those individuals have different needs than the individuals who are considered "treatment refractory" (meaning they are not responding to treatment).

Step 2: Assess Client's Concerns and Functional Deficits

After understanding the client's basic needs according to their phase of illness, it's important to not only assess the symptoms they are experiencing but to also assess a wide range of skills needed to function successfully in the community. The experience of having schizophrenia goes far beyond hallucinations and delusions and the other symptom criteria. **People with schizophrenia are known to have a variety of functional deficits, which result in significant disability**. Assessment should include cognitive skills, social skills, social functioning, medication adherence, money management, home maintenance, nutritious meal preparation, performance of inappropriate behaviors, and ability to function effectively in their environment. People with schizophrenia are often unreliable in describing their own functioning, so it's helpful to include information from multiple sources (e.g., case manager, family). With respect to functional deficits, a thorough assessment of what situations these deficits occur in, what triggers them, and what sort of function they perform (e.g., skipping their meds reduces unpleasant side effects) should follow. It is also important to consider whether personal factors affect the behaviors and deficits (e.g., personality characteristics, communication skills, sensory impairments) (Silverstein et al., 2006). These behavioral needs can then be combined with the other treatment planning information to select appropriate interventions to remediate areas of need.

Step 3: Discuss Client's Desires and Goals and Their Personal Resources

Because the deficits are so many, there is a tendency to focus on deficits and symptoms, but it's also important to focus on strengths and interests, as this will allow us to use the person's strengths and interests to compensate for weaknesses. An important point here is that treatment approaches are most effective when they account for the individual's unique pattern of strengths and needs. For that reason, treatment plans that are tailored specifically to *one* individual person and that include comprehensive services are more likely to result in significant functional improvements (reviewed in Silverstein et al., 2006).

Step 4: Construct the Treatment and Rehabilitation Plan

Because schizophrenia impacts not just brain functioning but functioning across the entire person's experience, extending from biological and neurophysiological impacts to cognitive, behavioral, family, and social (e.g., stigma, community availability of appropriate housing and medical care, etc.) impacts, it is imperative to have treatment approaches that target each of these areas and operate in concert. Unfortunately, until very recently, most treatment approaches have been developed in isolation. For example, psychological treatments aimed at changing how a person thinks about and reacts to hallucinations are developed separately from pharmacological treatments aimed at reducing hallucinatory experiences. **In selecting treatment interventions, the goal is to select interventions that will effectively reduce the problem behaviors identified in Step 2 with more appropriate, adaptable behaviors.** In other words, the goal is not to just control problem behaviors but to develop skills that can be used in the long term to decrease the likelihood of future hospitalization (Silverstein et al. 2006).

The following are interventions that are often available at the outpatient level of care (Silverstein et al., 2006), some of which are reviewed further below:

- Skills training
- Family intervention
- Supported employment
- Supported education

- Supported housing
- Individual or group psychotherapy
- Cognitive rehabilitation
- Integrated treatment for substance abuse and psychosis
- Assistance in accessing entitlements and healthcare
- Medication therapy
- Crisis assistance or respite care

Up to 60% of individuals can recover from schizophrenia when they are engaged in community-based rehabilitation programs with these types of intensive services. **In fact, when treatment goes beyond medication and emphasizes skills training that reduces disability and promotes community functioning, it is actually possible for individuals previously considered unresponsive to treatment to live in the community,** *even without medication* (reviewed in Silverstein et al., 2006). Further, young individuals experiencing their first or second psychotic episode can sometimes be successfully treated without medications, assuming they receive intensive interventions teaching other strategies to manage the symptoms and impairments associated with schizophrenia (reviewed in Silverstein et al., 2006). These facts about treating schizophrenia without medications are likely surprising to you, and indeed they are not well advertised. Certainly it's important to exercise caution in choosing not to pursue medication in treating schizophrenia, but it is also worth considering that there is evidence that some individuals with schizophrenia have become overly dependent on medication treatment, at the expense of other treatments that have equal or superior effectiveness (Silverstein et al., 2006).

Step 5: Establish Care Coordination and Implement Interventions

So, once a treatment plan has been made, it's probably got several different types of treatments or services on it. It's essential, then, that all the different treatment providers communicate among themselves. And that's tricky, especially at the outpatient level of care, because providers are not only separated geographically but they can also disagree philosophically and have a hard time working together. According to the recovery model, the treatment team includes not only all the professionals delivering services but also the individual diagnosed with schizophrenia, his or her legal representatives or substitute decision makers (those are people like parents, guardians, or even the mental health court if there is an inpatient or outpatient committal in process), and paraprofessionals who deliver services (like peer support workers). And while it's usually the *role* of case managers to coordinate all these treatment and service efforts, in practice, the treatments and services are usually delivered piece-meal rather than as a collaborative effort guided by an integrated team.

To address this limitation, Assertive Community Treatment (ACT) was developed. This is a treatment package designed to have a more collaborative treatment team, a systematic treatment plan, and intensive interventions, and it's been proven effective in preventing rehospitalization (reviewed in Silverstein et al., 2006). Part of what makes ACT so effective is the intensity of the services. Research indicates that consistent, intensive services improve outcomes for people with schizophrenia, whereas low intensity or intermittent treatment increases risk for relapse...by a lot (reviewed in Silverstein et al., 2006). In fact, people who receive ACT go back to the hospital less often, stay involved in their treatment services longer, show more stability in their living situation, and show improvements in symptoms and overall quality of life (reviewed in Silverstein et al., 2006). Unfortunately, only about 2% of the people who could really benefit from ACT are receiving it, in part because it requires a really healthy (and well financed...) public mental health system, which is hard to find (reviewed in Silverstein et al., 2006).

Step 6: Regularly Reevaluate Treatment Response and Modify Treatment Plan Accordingly

The final component of treatment planning is assessing how the person is responding to treatment over time and then modifying the treatment accordingly. This step is often skipped. Too often, we just implement the treatment plan and then assume it'll work. But it's important to actually check and see if the interventions are working to help people reach the goals that have been set. If medications aren't reducing symptoms, for example, the medications might be modified. Or if the person isn't responding to efforts to improve independent living skills, an alternative approach might be suggested.

Now that we know the basic process for creating a treatment plan, let's discuss more about the actual interventions that are commonly used to treat schizophrenia.

Chapter 17

Biological Treatments

Medications

Obviously, antipsychotic medications are approved to treat schizophrenia and other psychotic illnesses. They were developed to decrease hallucinations, delusional thinking, and paranoia and to increase the quality of life of people living with psychotic illnesses. Approximately 50% of people who take antipsychotics show remission of symptoms within three months of treatment, and up to 80% show remission within a year of treatment (reviewed in Combs & Mueser, 2007). Although not everyone who has schizophrenia needs or benefits from medication, for a lot of people, they play a major role in treating schizophrenia and keeping people well in the long term. For example, 70% of young people with schizophrenia who discontinue their medications relapse within a year, and 90% relapse within two years (reviewed in Silverstein et al., 2006). There are a couple of different kinds of antipsychotic medications, so let's discuss them.

First-Generation/Typical Antipsychotics

The first-generation antipsychotics (or "typical antipsychotics") were, naturally, the first ones developed. This generation includes haloperidol (Haldol), fluphenazine (Prolixin), trifluoperazine (Stelazine), and chlorpromazine (Thorazine). These medications work well at decreasing the frequency, intensity, and severity of auditory hallucinations and other positive symptoms and can greatly improve the daily life of a person with these debilitating symptoms. Recall from our chat about the dopamine hypothesis in Chapter 12 that there's a theory that schizophrenia is caused by having too much dopamine in the brain. So, inhibiting these receptors is thought to correct the symptoms of schizophrenia, and that's essentially how these first-generation drugs work. But blocking dopamine comes with some pretty nasty side effects (reviewed in Lambert & Kinsley, 2011), including restlessness, muscle stiffness, tremor, abnormal movements, and tardive dyskinesia. Tardive dyskinesia is a condition caused by using these medications that involves involuntary muscle movements (like facial tics and grimacing) that are disfiguring and usually permanent. Nobody wants that.

Second-Generation/Atypical Antipsychotics

Because the side effects of typical antipsychotics were so rough, a second generation of drugs was developed, including clozapine (Clozaril). Clozaril not only targets dopamine, as the first-generation drugs did, but it also works on serotonin, noradrenaline, and acetylcholine (reviewed in Lambert & Kinsley, 2011). As a result, drugs in this category treat a wider range of symptoms — not just hallucinations and delusions, but also some of the negative symptoms. And they also have fewer side effects, including decreased risk for tardive dyskinesia. But people who take Clozaril are at increased risk for a condition called agranulocytosis, which is a blood disorder resulting in a decrease in white blood cells, which help you fight infections. So people who take Clozaril get their blood drawn regularly to make sure they're okay in that regard.

Because Clozaril was so effective, attempts were made to replicate its effectiveness, with fewer side effects (and especially without that risk for agranulocytosis). Like Clozaril, this new class of drugs focused not only on dopamine but also on serotonin. This class includes medications like risperidone (Risperdal), olanzapine (Zyprexa), quetiapine (Seroquel), ziprasidone (Geodon), aripiprazole (Abilify), paliperidone (Invega), asenapine (Saphris), iloperidone (Fanapt), lurasidone (Latuda), brexpiprazole (Rexulti), and cariprazine (Vraylar). Because these drugs work on multiple neurotransmitters, they treat positive *and* negative symptoms without major motor side effects, but they have major problems with causing weight gain and increasing risk for diabetes and cardiovascular disease (reviewed in Lambert & Kinsley, 2011). The metabolic changes that cause such significant weight gain seem to be controlled by multiple genes (Zhang et al., 2016), and better understanding the genetic underpinnings may one day allow for better prediction of how a certain individual will respond to a given medication. Other side effects of atypical antipsychotics include resting tremor, gait changes, dry mouth, increased cholesterol, drowsiness, increased heart rate, dizziness, lightheadedness, increased appetite, restlessness, decreased libido, menstruation irregularity, skin rash, increased sensitivity to the sun, muscle stiffness (especially risperidone), thickening of the tongue, twisting of the neck, arching of the back, and rolling up of the eyes. Yikes.

Because of the risk for agranulocytosis and because newer drugs were developed that did not carry that risk, doctors stopped prescribing Clozaril as much. However, recent research suggests individuals treated with Clozaril live longer (i.e., have a lower long-term mortality rate) than individuals treated with other antipsychotics, so consideration is returning to using Clozaril (Vermeulen et al., 2018).

Medication Concerns

Unfortunately, despite all the research that has gone into developing antipsychotics, there are still a lot of people who don't respond to antipsychotic medications. People who have an earlier age of onset of their illness tend to have higher rates of nonresponsiveness to antipsychotic medications (Samara, Nikolakopoulou, Salanti, & Leucht, 2018).

And although medications continue to be developed, there are some opinions that their effectiveness has stalled (e.g., Lambert & Kinsley, 2011). Psychiatric medications change the concentration of neurotransmitters but not the structure of the pathways they operate on. In other words, they change the number of cars on the road, but not where the road goes. If the messages are being routed incorrectly (the road is going to the wrong destination), the medication will have limited efficacy. Connections between the hippocampus and several other brain areas (anterior cingulate cortex, caudate nucleus, auditory cortex, calcarine sulcus) are particularly responsive to antipsychotic medications and are especially important in predicting response to antipsychotic medications (Kraguljac et al., 2016).

With the cognitive deficits associated with schizophrenia, a lot of people have trouble remembering to take their medications or they don't have the insight to understand medications are needed or helpful. On top of that, medications tend to be fairly nonspecific and the side effects decrease *willingness* to take them. In fact, as many as 75% of individuals with schizophrenia don't take their medications as prescribed (reviewed in Silverstein et al., 2006). Also, many medications create confusion and other cognitive deficits. So it's important to balance the utility of medications in reducing symptoms with the energy and cognition needed to function effectively in the community and benefit from other treatment services (Silverstein et al., 2006). For that reason, many individuals function best with lower medication doses that actually allow them to be more alert, even if that means they continue to experience some psychotic symptoms (reviewed in Silverstein et al., 2006). In that context, it's not surprising that the combination of medications plus a range of psychosocial interventions tends to produce better outcomes for individuals with schizophrenia than medications alone (reviewed in Silverstein et al., 2006).

Other Biological Treatments

Medications aren't the only biological treatment available for treating schizophrenia. Transcranial magnetic stimulation is an intervention in which magnetic fields are used to repeatedly stimulate nerve cells in the brain. This suppresses auditory hallucinations in individuals with schizophrenia, and the results last several months (reviewed in Lambert & Kinsley, 2011). Really recent research is also showing that direct stimulation of the prefrontal cortex in schizophrenia with transcranial direct current stimulation shows promise for treating negative symptoms in schizophrenia (Palm et al., 2016). Electroconvulsive therapy is similar, except electrical rather than magnetic stimulation is used, which induces seizures and requires anesthesia. Sounds scary, but it's actually reasonably safe these days. This treatment can be effective for treating catatonia in schizophrenia.

Chapter 18

Psychosocial Treatments

Medications can be helpful in reducing the positive and negative symptoms of schizophrenia but do little to address the other deficits that accompany the diagnosis, such as impairments in social skills and living skills. These impairments don't seem to be caused by the same neurophysiological abnormalities that cause the specific symptoms of schizophrenia and rather seem to come from (1) the effects of living with schizophrenia (e.g., how it affects the person socially and cognitively) and (2) the myriad developmental difficulties the person experienced before they ever developed schizophrenia (reviewed in Silverstein et al., 2006).

It's important to address these skill deficits in addition to the positive symptoms of psychosis because **the symptoms of schizophrenia themselves don't appear to be significantly tied to how well a person functions in their life and in the community** (i.e., a person can still function well, despite having hallucinations or delusions). **Instead, deficits in *skills* have been consistently shown to compromise functioning** (reviewed in Silverstein et al., 2006). Further, the stronger a person's social skills and independent living skills are, the more likely they are to (1) stick to an outpatient treatment program after discharging from the hospital and (2) live successfully in the community without relapsing (reviewed in Silverstein et al., 2006). For these reasons, significantly better outcomes are seen with the combination of medications *plus* psychosocial interventions (i.e., the interventions that address personal psychological experience and interaction with the environment; this includes psychotherapy, case management, self-help and support groups, supported employment services, etc.). These improved outcomes include a 20% lower risk of relapse over a 12-month period.

So, ultimately, the goal of treatment (at least from a recovery or psychiatric rehabilitation model) is to help a person function effectively in the community and live a meaningful life. It's assumed (Silverstein et al., 2006) this goal depends on three main things:

1. The person's individual characteristics, such as their particular symptoms, their cognitive abilities, and their personality
2. The community's characteristics, such as whether knowledge of a public transportation system is expected, whether there are high crime rates, or how many social services are available
3. How supportive the environment is, including the individual's family and friends, professional supports, and neighbors, coworkers, and community members

That information needs to be incorporated into the treatment plan in determining which of the following interventions might be needed to optimize community functioning. Now that we've established how psychosocial treatments can be helpful in general, let's discuss some specific interventions.

Skills Training

As we've discussed, if a person with schizophrenia is going to function successfully in the community, they need to have a certain set of skills, and these skills were often never developed because they were so young when they developed schizophrenia or the skills were lost when the person developed schizophrenia.

In developing a plan to rehabilitate skill deficits, it's important to distinguish between *skill* deficits and *performance* deficits. A skill deficit reflects a person's complete inability to complete the activity. For example, I don't have the slightest idea *how* to change the oil in my car myself, so this is a skill deficit. A performance deficit, however, reflects a person's inability or failure to *use* a skill in real time. For example, assuming I know *how* to change the oil in my car myself, my failure to actually *do* it on a regular basis reflects a performance deficit. Individuals with schizophrenia often are able to demonstrate skills on lab tests that they don't demonstrate in their real lives. So they might be able to set up a budget in an office or treatment environment but then be unable to manage their money in their real lives. Put another way, there's a difference between *impairment* (poor performance on lab tests) and *disability* (reduced real-world functioning) (e.g., Silverstein et al., 2006). Distinguishing between these components helps direct treatment efforts to either teaching the skill itself or teaching how and when to implement the skill.

Cognitive Skills

In Chapter 1, we talked a lot about the cognitive impairments associated with schizophrenia. This includes things like problems with attention, memory, and abstract reasoning. Medications, including the newest atypical antipsychotics, don't do much to improve these cognitive deficits and in many cases can actually make cognitive skills worse (reviewed in Silverstein et al., 2006). For that reason, cognitive training is a preferred method to improve cognitive functioning or to at least help people figure out how to compensate for their deficits.

Cognitive training was born out of treatment for traumatic brain injuries and is designed to help people improve attention and problem solving, with more recently developed treatments also focusing on motivation, the ability to engage in tasks, and beliefs in your ability to accomplish tasks or succeed in certain situations (reviewed in Silverstein et al., 2006). It's proven to improve cognition in schizophrenia and even has at least a small positive impact on negative symptoms (Cella, Preti, Edwards, Dow, & Wykes, 2017). Cognitive training also helps people monitor their ideas and speech more effectively and improve how well they coordinate their movements and thoughts (reviewed in Lambert & Kinsley, 2011).

A subset of this broader focus on cognitive skills is problem-solving skills. Another unfortunate side effect of having schizophrenia is that the person's problem-solving skills can become impaired. Instruction in the basic five-step model of problem-solving (identify the problem, brainstorm solutions, evaluate solutions, choose one to implement, evaluate outcome) can greatly improve outcomes.

A specific area of cognitive training that's relevant for schizophrenia is in *social* cognition, which refers to how we interpret, use, and apply social information. This includes interpreting emotions (i.e., emotion perception), understanding what other people are thinking and how their thoughts differ from ours (i.e., theory of mind), and explaining what causes events (i.e., attributional style; e.g., do the events in my life happen by coincidence, accident, or my own doing?). Social cognition training significantly improves theory of mind and emotion recognition, but current evidence is less clear about whether it changes attributional style (Grant, Lawrence, Preti, Wykes, & Cella, 2017).

Cognitive training isn't just helpful for people with schizophrenia who have had cognitive deficits for years, but also for people who are at risk for developing schizophrenia. Training that works on how your brain interprets information you're hearing improves memory for words and other verbal information. This is important because people who are risk for developing schizophrenia tend to have difficulties with that type of verbal memory, and that difficulty actually predicts who will go on to have schizophrenia (Loewy et al., 2016).

The next level of cognitive training is *meta*cognitive training. If cognitive training is training your brain to think better, metacognitive training is training your brain to think *about* thinking better. Metacognition is a skill we use all the time to identify what we're thinking, recognize if we're overreacting or taking something personally, and try to think more rationally -- we're thinking about the thoughts we're having. Metacognitive training in schizophrenia actually improves delusions and positive symptoms at least a little bit and is really helpful for getting people to understand and participate in this type of training (reviewed in Silverstein et al., 2006).

Besides directly targeting cognition with these types of cognitive training, cognition can also improve with less direct interventions, like exercise. Just like with everyone else, people with schizophrenia who exercise more see larger benefits -- in this case, more improvements in their cognition (Firth et al., 2016). This includes improvements in working memory (keeping information in their head while they solve a problem or complete a task), social cognition (the way we perceive, interpret, and understand social information), attention (but not processing speed), memory, and reasoning (Firth et al., 2016).

Living Skills

Just as medications don't do much for the cognitive deficits in schizophrenia, they also don't improve deficits in community-based living skills (reviewed in Silverstein et al., 2006). Because of the onset of schizophrenia in early adulthood, some people never develop the skills associated with living independently. They're far too busy during their early 20s fighting off the hallucinations and delusions to be worried about budgeting and dishwashing. And other folks with schizophrenia lose these skills along the way as the illness takes hold. But they need these basic skills to be able to function effectively in the real world because deficits in independent living skills cause major stress and make it much more likely a person is going to have a psychotic relapse (reviewed in Silverstein et al., 2006). In fact, deficits in this area can contribute to homelessness, which is a major problem in schizophrenia, as between 10% and 20% of people with schizophrenia are homeless. In the category of living skills are skills such as basic healthcare (using Band-Aids, taking Tylenol, knowing when to make medical appointments), grooming and hygiene, keeping a daily schedule, housekeeping, making nutritious meals, managing personal funds, and using public transportation and other public resources. When people can perform these behaviors well, they are prepared to function more effectively as members of the community.

Social Skills

A specialized area of cognitive functioning is processing social information. Individuals with schizophrenia have deficits in perceiving, interpreting, understanding, and using social information. This includes skills such as perceiving emotional and social cues (e.g., facial expressions, body language), predicting others' intentions and motivations, and having empathy. There are obvious parallels to autism here, especially for people with high-functioning autism and high-functioning psychotic disorders (like schizotypal personality disorder). This may relate to their shared genetic risk (reviewed in Murray et al., 2017). Despite the similarities in functioning, the social cognitive deficits in autism and psychosis have different brain mechanisms (Stanfield et al., 2017), pointing to different causes that ultimately lead to the same outcome.

Social skills training is an important component of an overall skills training package for schizophrenia. Schizophrenia changes the way people think about social information, which then affects how they behave socially. For example, people with schizophrenia have more difficulty recognizing facial expressions and actually tend to interpret *neutral* facial expressions as *threatening* [Side note: this is the same error a lot of us make with RBF, except much more intense]. You can imagine, then, if they're seeing a whole bunch of threatening faces around why they would become withdrawn or maybe even hostile. So there are two major treatment goals here -- one is to help them *interpret* that social information more accurately (which we discussed above, under Cognitive Skills), and the other is to *respond* to that social information more effectively, which is where social skills training comes in. Social skills training helps them rehabilitate some of the basic social skills that get taken by the illness. This includes things like starting a conversation, asking for things you need, maintaining friendships, saying no to a request, and developing appropriate intimacy in relationships.

Unfortunately, social skills training is often executed poorly. Most often, it involves teaching clients *about* the skills without ever *rehearsing* or *practicing* the skills. Correctly-implemented social skills training is almost entirely roleplays because the behavioral rehearsal has been determined to be the most important training element. Part of the reason this rehearsal is important is because the cognitive deficits of schizophrenia interfere with their ability to apply information to new situations (reviewed in Combs & Mueser, 2007), so teaching the skills in the specific situation in which they will be used is critical. When done well, social skills training helps people with schizophrenia improve their functioning in relationships, as you'd expect, but it goes far beyond that. Social skills training can actually reduce how frequently people return to the hospital and lessen how severe their symptoms are (reviewed in Silverstein et al., 2006). Pretty cool.

Occupational Skills

Although many people with schizophrenia *want* to work, few do. In fact, only 10% to 30% of individuals with schizophrenia are employed, and only a handful of those are able to maintain consistent employment (reviewed in Silverstein et al., 2006). Employment is important in the treatment plan for schizophrenia because people with schizophrenia who are employed tend to fare better in terms of the severity of their illness and their quality of life is better (reviewed in Silverstein et al., 2006). But the symptoms of schizophrenia and the cognitive impairment that comes along with schizophrenia make it hard to work. In fact, neurocognitive deficits are a significant predictor of occupational deficits in schizophrenia (McGurk et al., 2017). So, getting a person to return to work takes effort from the treatment team (including the person with schizophrenia).

There are a couple of approaches to enhancing employment opportunities for people with schizophrenia -- one is vocational rehabilitation (voc rehab), which you might be familiar with, and the other is supported employment, which might be new to you. Here are the main differences (from Silverstein et al., 2006). In voc rehab, the jobs are held by the program, whereas in supported employment, the jobs are held by the client. In this way, supported employment is no different from what is happening in your life -- you hold your job, and it is your responsibility. Also, supported employment is more integrated with the person's treatment plan than voc rehab tends to be, and the goal is to place people in competitive employment, with as much support as needed, for as long as needed rather than place them in sheltered employment.

The values of supported employment are in line with the recovery model (Wehman, 2012). Supported employment presumes everyone, regardless of their disability, has the capability and right to work in regular community businesses earning the same wages and benefits of other people performing the same or similar jobs. The focus is much more on abilities, strengths, and interests rather than disabilities. If people choose and manage their employment and how they are supported with their employment, they tend to be more satisfied with their career. Relationships are important in supported employment, and it focuses on assisting people in assembling a team of supportive individuals to help them achieve their ambitions.

Once people are placed in a job, they need assistance with various occupational skills. This ranges from things like arriving to work on time, selecting appropriate workplace attire, maintaining appropriate grooming and hygiene standards for work, staying on task, following directions, asking for assistance, managing relationships with coworkers and supervisors, navigating pay and benefits, etc. Supported employment specialists (or other employment specialists if the person is not specifically receiving supported employment services) help with this skill development.

Unfortunately, even with supported employment services, the rates of competitive employment in schizophrenia are low. Only a third of people with schizophrenia work more than 20 hours a week. And while most full-time working Americans work 50 weeks per year, most people with schizophrenia work fewer than 15 weeks per year, and they earn only about $1000 per year (reviewed in Silverstein et al., 2006).

Other Skills

There are a host of other skill deficits that individuals with schizophrenia have, either because they never developed the skills or because they lost them as the illness developed. In developing a treatment plan, it's critical to assess which of these areas might be impaired and to then assign interventions to remediate the deficits so the person can function more effectively in their environment. Some examples include managing medications (e.g., knowing how to fill up a med cassette, knowing when to request refills, taking medications at prescribed times) and managing the illness more generally (e.g., identifying warning signs of relapse, knowing what symptoms are persistent, understanding how symptoms relate to functioning, using coping skills and other interventions to manage symptoms, managing medication side effects, etc.). In addition, leisure skills (e.g., developing adaptive hobbies and leisure interests to challenge the mind and provide a source of pleasure and socialization) are an often neglected area of skill development.

Psychotherapy

Despite taking medications to control long-term symptoms of psychosis, many individuals continue to experience hallucinations and delusions that don't respond to medications. Cognitive-behavioral therapy is the front-line psychotherapy for most mental health conditions, from depression to anxiety to insomnia to chronic pain. There's also a version of cognitive-behavioral therapy that is specially designed for psychosis.

Just like in other versions of CBT, the goal of CBT for psychosis is to challenge how the person interprets events and experiences in their life and then develop alternative, more evidence-based interpretations. When this is applied to schizophrenia, that takes the form of trying to develop non-paranoid or non-delusional interpretations of events and coming up with less stressful ways of explaining hallucinatory experiences.

Here's another example of CBT in action. When we don't think we'll be able to perform a behavior well, most of us don't bother even starting. If I don't think I can ever successfully make a molten lava cake, I won't bother researching and experimenting to learn how to do it. This is true in schizophrenia as well, except they have even more negative thoughts that interfere with doing the things they need to do. This is compounded by negative symptoms and compromises their ability to function well in their environment (Campellone et al., 2016). So targeting those beliefs about the ability to successfully achieve goals are a good CBT intervention, as it would be for anyone who has those beliefs.

CBT for psychosis also makes use of classic CBT interventions used in other mental health conditions, like scheduling activities, rewarding yourself for doing pleasurable activities, etc. What's really neat is that because the same basic CBT principles are used in CBT for psychosis and CBT for everything else, the person already has the skills needed to treat the ancillary, comorbid conditions that accompany schizophrenia - things like social anxiety, substance use, and depression.

CBT for psychosis has been shown to be effective in treating positive psychotic symptoms (Tarrier, 2008), including in reducing delusional thinking, paranoia, distress from hallucinations, and even negative symptoms (reviewed in Silverstein et al., 2006). **CBT for psychosis is also being shown to be effective early in the development of schizophrenia and has shown some benefit in preventing symptoms from escalating into a full-blown psychotic illness, in reducing or preventing the need for antipsychotic medications, and in reducing symptoms during the prodromal period of the illness** (reviewed in Tarrier, 2008). The ability to think about thoughts and confront uncomfortable thoughts, as is a focus of cognitive-behavioral therapy, may actually affect the effectiveness of all the other treatments and services the person is receiving (reviewed in Silverstein et al., 2006).

Unfortunately, specialized CBT for psychosis isn't widely available. Because of the supply-demand issue, research is being conducted to determine the minimum number of sessions needed to achieve the impressive outcomes associated with CBT for psychosis. Usually, at least 16 sessions are recommended, but preliminary evidence suggests fewer sessions might be sufficient (Hazell, Hayward, Cavanagh, & Strauss, 2016). Jury's still out.

We know CBT for psychosis is effective, but what about other types of therapy? The evidence is mixed. The most caution should be exercised with using psychodynamic therapy to treat schizophrenia. There is some evidence that some people with schizophrenia can actually get *worse* with psychodynamic treatment, so this should only be attempted with *stable* individuals and by really experienced therapists (reviewed in Silverstein et al., 2006). For now, CBT for psychosis is the most evidence-based psychotherapy for psychotic conditions.

Substance Use

As we discussed earlier, substance abuse is widespread among people with schizophrenia, so substance use services are another important psychosocial intervention for people with schizophrenia. This is in part because of the high rates of substance use in this population and also to the association between substance use and relapse. For example, **using drugs or alcohol *doubles* the rate of relapse over a one- to two-year period in schizophrenia** (reviewed in Silverstein et al., 2006). It also interferes with rehabilitation and recovery from schizophrenia (reviewed in Silverstein et al., 2006). Traditional 12-step programs can be effective for people with schizophrenia, but there are also more specialized programs to treat substance use in schizophrenia, and current best practice standards involve treating schizophrenia and substance use together by the same treatment team (Silverstein et al., 2006).

Family Interventions

In treating a person with schizophrenia, it's critical to involve the family. The family often makes up a massive portion of the person's support network and as such plays a huge role in maintaining wellness. Plus, between 25% and 60% of people with schizophrenia live at home with their relatives, with even more people relying on caregiver support without living at home (reviewed in Combs & Mueser, 2007).

When families receive education about the person's illness, are taught communication skills to reduce criticism, and receive their own supports, this has positive outcomes not only for the family but also for the person with schizophrenia. For the family, they feel more supported by the treatment team, learn more about schizophrenia treatment and rehabilitation, improve their own coping abilities, and reduce the stress and self-blame that's so common in supporting a person with a disability (reviewed in Silverstein et al., 2006). And for the person with schizophrenia, when their family receives interventions, they relapse less often, adhere to their treatment plans better, and return to the hospital less often (Sin et al., 2017; and reviewed in Silverstein et al., 2006). Often, these types of family interventions are delivered in weekly hour-long group sessions with other family members (Sin et al., 2017).

Chapter 19

Inpatient Services

Almost all of the services described so far can be delivered in inpatient or outpatient settings, though usually they're delivered at the outpatient level of care. About 25% of all psychiatric hospital beds are filled by people with schizophrenia (Combs & Mueser, 2007), making effective inpatient treatment of schizophrenia critical. Inpatient treatment programs are most often short-term (e.g., 3 days) to stabilize medications and return to the community. But long-term inpatient programs exist for people who are not responding to typical treatments and continue to have major functional impairment that results in legal charges or substantial risk of harm to self or others. Although many of these individuals are considered "treatment refractory," meaning they don't respond to typical treatments, they can make substantial improvements in specially-designed inpatient programs based on the principles of psychiatric rehabilitation.

There are different versions of this type of specially-designed inpatient program, but social learning programs are perhaps the most widely used. In these programs, the hospital environment is extremely positive and focused on teaching and coaching so the clients (often called "participants") learn the skills they need to be successful once they get back into the community. There's often a point system so they earn certain privileges and are reinforced for learning these skills, and there's a focus on finding opportunities to practice the skills in the real world (because what good is it if you can use the archaic washing machine in the hospital but have no idea how to use the fancy machines at the local laundromat?).

In other words, continuing to rely solely on medications is ineffective in reducing recurrent rehospitalization, but teaching people skills to live a productive, meaningful life despite having persistent symptoms can result in successful discharge from long-term treatment programs (reviewed in Silverstein et al., 2006), especially when combined with careful aftercare plans that gradually reduce the intensity of services. Inpatient programs of this type go through the same six-step treatment planning process outlined above, but they do it iteratively at regular intervals until the client meets the established treatment goals.

SUMMARY

Congratulations! You made it to the end. Evidence shows reviewing newly-created memories helps them sink in deeper, and you probably want to make sure you remember what you just spent all this time reading. So let's recap based on the objectives of this book.

Objective 1: Distinguish between positive and negative psychotic symptoms

What we call "schizophrenia" represents an expert consensus regarding a group of psychological experiences that tend to cluster together, but there aren't any symptoms that are unique to schizophrenia. In other words, it's not that a person has various psychotic symptoms that results in the diagnosis; rather, when the symptoms and their associated impairment rise above a certain arbitrary threshold, a psychotic disorder diagnosis is considered. Symptoms are clustered into positive symptoms (things that are added to the usual experience, like hallucinations and delusions) and negative symptoms (things that are missing from the usual experience, like emotional expression and motivation).

Objective 2: Identify the major mental health conditions that co-occur with schizophrenia

People with schizophrenia experience higher rates of depression, anxiety, substance use, and suicide than the general population, and they also have a host of physical health problems that result in their having a shorter life expectancy. Treating schizophrenia requires considering these comorbid conditions as well.

Objective 3: Name at least two factors that increase risk for schizophrenia

The current best explanation of schizophrenia is that it is a neurodevelopmental disorder with signs beginning in gestation. Men tend to develop schizophrenia earlier in life than women, but late adolescence and early adulthood is the key time for the acute onset of the illness. This acute onset is preceded by a period of months to years of prodromal symptoms. Certain genetic markers, gestational problems, childhood trauma, living in an urban environment, and using cannabis increase risk for schizophrenia. Schizophrenia is associated with differences in how the brain is structured (e.g., larger ventricles, less volume in the cortex) and how it functions (e.g., problems transmitting and coordinating messages across the brain). An early hypothesis that schizophrenia was caused by excess dopamine has been replaced by hypotheses that schizophrenia is associated with dysfunction in multiple neurotransmitter systems in the brain and is caused by genes that affect how the brain develops.

Objective 4: Explain how cannabis use affects risk for schizophrenia Cannabis use doubles the risk for schizophrenia. It's just that simple.

Objective 5: Describe the recovery model of schizophrenia

The medical model treats schizophrenia as though it were a physical condition and targets primarily the *symptoms* of schizophrenia, with medication being the key treatment intervention. The recovery model is a much broader perspective, with a focus on reducing disability and leading a productive, meaningful, fulfilling life. The psychiatric rehabilitation model is based on this and considers how schizophrenia develops, is experienced, and is expressed. It focuses on real-world community functioning, with multiple treatment modalities being used in a coordinated and integrated fashion. By this model, treatment planning is collaborative and accounts for the person's disabilities as well as their strengths, preferences, and goals. Medications continue to be an important treatment intervention, but skills training is an important adjunct because symptoms of schizophrenia themselves don't appear to be significantly tied to how well a person functions in their life and in the community; instead, deficits in skills have been consistently shown to compromise functioning. Training in cognitive skills, social skills, living skills, occupational skills, etc. are all necessary treatment targets, and adding in family services enhances treatment effectiveness. CBT for psychosis has been shown to be effective in treating psychotic symptoms as well and early research suggests it might actually reduce the need for medications.

Objective 6: Identify the major classes of medication effective in treating schizophrenia

Schizophrenia is treated with "typical antipsychotics" and "atypical antipsychotics." Typical antipsychotics have lots of nasty side effects, especially on motor functioning, and they reduce positive symptoms by working in the dopamine system. Atypical antipsychotics have a better side effect profile and work on a larger network of neurotransmitters.

Objective 7: Explain the importance of family support in treating a person with schizophrenia

People with schizophrenia are often cared for by their families, and many of them live at home. When their families receive treatment alongside them, this improves outcomes for the person with schizophrenia.

There you have it. By completing this book, you now know the basics about what schizophrenia looks like, how it affects a person's life, what causes it, and how it's treated. Now you have some initial information to begin supporting those around you who might be experiencing psychotic symptoms, or maybe you have a better understanding of what exactly is happening to you. Remember, this book covered "averages" and "typical" experiences, but the experience of having and living with schizophrenia is different for everyone. Recovery is absolutely possible.

REFERENCES

1. Bailey, T., Alvarez-Jimenez, M., Garcia-Sanchez, A. M., Hulbert, C., Barlow, E., & Bendall, S. (2018). Childhood trauma is associated with severity of hallucinations and delusions in psychotic disorders: A systematic review and meta-analysis. *Schizophrenia Bulletin, 44*(5), 1111-1122. doi:10.1093/schbul/sbx161

2. Baumeister, D., Sedgwick, O., Howes, O., & Peters, E. (2017). Auditory verbal hallucinations and continuum models of psychosis: A systematic review of the healthy voice-hearer literature. *Clinical Psychology Review, 51*, 125-141. doi:10.1016/j.cpr.2016.10.010

3. Bhatia, M. S., Goyal, A., Saha, R., & Doval, N. (2017). Psychogenic polydipsia - Management challenges. *Shanghai Archives of Psychiatry, 29*(3), 180-183.

4. Bohlken, M. M., Brouwer, R. M., Mandl, R. C., Kahn, R. S., & Pol, H. E. (2016). Genetic variation in schizophrenia liability is shared with intellectual ability and brain structure. *Schizophrenia Bulletin, 42*(5), 1167-1175. doi:10.1093/schbul/sbw034

5. Campellone, T. R., Sanchez, A. H., & Kring, A. M. (2016). Defeatist performance beliefs, negative symptoms, and functional outcome in schizophrenia: A meta-analytic review. *Schizophrenia Bulletin, 42*(6), 1343-1352. doi:10.1093/schbul/sbw026

6. Carrión, R. E., Auther, A. M., Mclaughlin, D., Olsen, R., Addington, J., Bearden, C. E., . . . Cornblatt, B. A. (2018). The global functioning: Social and role scales — Further validation in a large sample of adolescents and young adults at clinical high risk for psychosis. *Schizophrenia Bulletin.* doi:10.1093/schbul/sby126

7. Cella, M., Preti, A., Edwards, C., Dow, T., & Wykes, T. (2017). Cognitive remediation for negative symptoms of schizophrenia: A network meta-analysis. *Clinical Psychology Review, 52*, 43-51. doi:10.1016/j.cpr.2016.11.009

8. Coid, J. W., Ullrich, S., Bebbington, P., Fazel, S., & Keers, R. (2016). Paranoid ideation and violence: Meta-analysis of individual subject data of 7 population surveys. *Schizophrenia Bulletin, 42*(4), 907-915. doi:10.1093/schbul/sbw006

9. Combs, D. R., & Mueser, K. T. (2007). Schizophrenia. In *Adult Psychopathology and Diagnosis* (5th ed., pp. 234-285). Hoboken, NJ: John Wiley & Sons.

10. *Diagnostic and Statistical Manual of Mental Disorders* (5th ed.). (2013). Arlington, VA: American Psychiatric Association.

11. Dwyer, D. B., Cabral, C., Kambeitz-Ilankovic, L., Sanfelici, R., Kambeitz, J., Calhoun, V., . . . Koutsouleris, N. (2018). Brain subtyping enhances the neuroanatomical discrimination of schizophrenia. *Schizophrenia Bulletin, 44*(5), 1060-1069. doi:10.1093/schbul/sby008

12. Firth, J., Stubbs, B., Rosenbaum, S., Vancampfort, D., Malchow, B., Schuch, F., . . . Yung, A. R. (2016). Aerobic exercise improves cognitive functioning in people with schizophrenia: A systematic review and meta-analysis. *Schizophrenia Bulletin*. doi:10.1093/schbul/sbw115

13. Fusar-Poli, P., Cappucciati, M., Rutigliano, G., Heslin, M., Stahl, D., Brittenden, Z., . . . Carpenter, W. T. (2016). Diagnostic stability of ICD/DSM first episode psychosis diagnoses: Meta-analysis. *Schizophrenia Bulletin, 42*(6), 1395-1406. doi:10.1093/schbul/sbw020

14. Gibson, L. E., Alloy, L. B., & Ellman, L. M. (2016). Trauma and the psychosis spectrum: A review of symptom specificity and explanatory mechanisms. *Clinical Psychology Review, 49*, 92-105. doi:10.1016/j.cpr.2016.08.003

15. Gold, J. M., Robinson, B., Leonard, C. J., Hahn, B., Chen, S., McMahon, R. P., & Luck, S. J. (2017). Selective attention, working

memory, and executive function as potential independent sources of cognitive dysfunction in schizophrenia. *Schizophrenia Bulletin*, 44(6), 1227-1234. doi:10.1093/schbul/sbx155

16. Grant, N., Lawrence, M., Preti, A., Wykes, T., & Cella, M. (2017). Social cognition interventions for people with schizophrenia: A systematic review focussing on methodological quality and intervention modality. *Clinical Psychology Review*, 56, 55-64. doi:10.1016/j.cpr.2017.06.001

17. Hardy, A., Emsley, R., Freeman, D., Bebbington, P., Garety, P. A., Kuipers, E. E., . . . Fowler, D. (2016). Psychological mechanisms mediating effects between trauma and psychotic symptoms: The role of affect regulation, intrusive trauma memory, beliefs, and depression. *Schizophrenia Bulletin*, 42(Suppl 1). doi:10.1093/schbul/sbv175

18. Hazell, C. M., Hayward, M., Cavanagh, K., & Strauss, C. (2016). A systematic review and meta-analysis of low intensity CBT for psychosis. *Clinical Psychology Review*, 45, 183-192. doi:10.1016/j.cpr.2016.03.004

19. Isvoranu, A., Borkulo, C. D., Boyette, L., Wigman, J. T., Vinkers, C. H., & Borsboom, D. (2016). A network approach to psychosis: pathways between childhood trauma and psychotic symptoms. *Schizophrenia Bulletin*, 43(1), 187-196. doi:10.1093/schbul/sbw055

20. Isvoranu, A., Borsboom, D., Os, J. V., & Guloksuz, S. (2016). A network approach to environmental impact in psychotic disorder: brief theoretical framework. *Schizophrenia Bulletin*, 42(4), 870-873. doi:10.1093/schbul/sbw049

21. Kelleher, I., Cederlöf, M., Kuja-Halkola, R., Larsson, H., Sjölander, A., Östberg, P., . . . Lichtenstein, P. (2017). Psychotic experiences in adolescence and later risk of suicidal behavior and substance use in a Swedish longitudinal cohort. *Schizophrenia Bulletin*, 43(Suppl_1). doi:10.1093/schbul/sbx021.024

22. Klauser, P., Baker, S. T., Cropley, V. L., Bousman, C., Fornito, A., Cocchi, L., . . . Zalesky, A. (2016). White matter disruptions in

schizophrenia are spatially widespread and topologically converge on brain network hubs. *Schizophrenia Bulletin.* doi:10.1093/schbul/sbw100

23. Kraguljac, N. V., White, D. M., Hadley, N., Hadley, J. A., Hoef, L. V., Davis, E., & Lahti, A. C. (2016). Aberrant hippocampal connectivity in unmedicated patients with schizophrenia and effects of antipsychotic medication: A longitudinal resting state functional MRI study. *Schizophrenia Bulletin*, 42(4), 1046-1055. doi:10.1093/schbul/sbv228

24. Krystal, J. H., Murray, J. D., Chekroud, A. M., Corlett, P. R., Yang, G., Wang, X., & Anticevic, A. (2017). Computational psychiatry and the challenge of schizophrenia. *Schizophrenia Bulletin*, 43(3), 473-475. doi:10.1093/schbul/sbx025

25. Lambert, K., & Kinsley, C. H. (2011). *Clinical Neuroscience.* New York: Oxford University Press.

26. Leung, A., & Chue, P. (2000). Sex differences in schizophrenia, a review of the literature. *Acta Psychiatrica Scandinavica, 101*(401), 3-38. doi:10.1111/j.0065-1591.2000.0ap25.x

27. Li, T., Wang, Q., Zhang, J., Rolls, E. T., Yang, W., Palaniyappan, L., . . . Feng, J. (2016). Brain-wide analysis of functional connectivity in first-episode and chronic stages of schizophrenia. *Schizophrenia Bulletin.* doi:10.1093/schbul/sbw099

28. Loewy, R., Fisher, M., Schlosser, D. A., Biagianti, B., Stuart, B., Mathalon, D. H., & Vinogradov, S. (2016). Intensive auditory cognitive training improves verbal memory in adolescents and young adults at clinical high risk for psychosis. *Schizophrenia Bulletin*, 42(Suppl 1). doi:10.1093/schbul/sbw009

29. Loranger, A. W. (1984). Sex difference in age at onset of schizophrenia. *Journal of Clinical Psychopharmacology*, 4(4), 236. doi:10.1097/00004714-198408000-00033

30. Lysaker, P. H., Gagen, E., Wright, A., Vohs, J. L., Kukla, M., Yanos, P. T., & Hasson-Ohayon, I. (2018). Metacognitive deficits predict impaired insight in schizophrenia across symptom profiles: a latent

class analysis. *Schizophrenia Bulletin, 45*(1), 48-56. doi:10.1093/schbul/sby142

31. Marconi, A., Forti, M. D., Lewis, C. M., Murray, R. M., & Vassos, E. (2016). Meta-analysis of the association between the level of cannabis use and risk of psychosis. *Schizophrenia Bulletin, 42*(5), 1262-1269. doi:10.1093/schbul/sbw003

32. Mcgrath, J., Saha, S., Welham, J., Saadi, O. E., Maccauley, C., & Chant, D. (2004). A systematic review of the incidence of schizophrenia: The distribution of rates and the influence of sex, urbanicity, migrant status and methodology. *BMC Medicine, 2*(1). doi:10.1186/1741-7015-2-13

33. McGurk, S. R., Drake, R. E., Xie, H., Riley, J., Milfort, R., Hale, T. W., & Frey, W. (2017). Cognitive predictors of work among social security disability insurance beneficiaries with psychiatric disorders enrolled in IPS supported employment. *Schizophrenia Bulletin, 44*(1), 32-37. doi:10.1093/schbul/sbx115

34. Murray, R. M., Bhavsar, V., Tripoli, G., & Howes, O. (2017). 30 years on: How the neurodevelopmental hypothesis of schizophrenia morphed into the developmental risk factor model of psychosis. *Schizophrenia Bulletin, 43*(6), 1190-1196. doi:10.1093/schbul/sbx121

35. Newbury, J., Arseneault, L., Caspi, A., Moffitt, T. E., Odgers, C. L., & Fisher, H. L. (2016). Why are children in urban neighborhoods at increased risk for psychotic symptoms? Findings from a UK longitudinal cohort study. *Schizophrenia Bulletin, 42*(6), 1372-1383. *doi:10.1093/schbul/sbw052*

36. Newbury, J., Arseneault, L., Caspi, A., Moffitt, T. E., Odgers, C. L., & Fisher, H. L. (2017). Cumulative effects of neighborhood social adversity and personal crime victimization on adolescent psychotic experiences. *Schizophrenia Bulletin, 44*(2), 348-358. doi:10.1093/schbul/sbx060

37. Ng, S., Yeung, C., & Gao, S. (2019). A concise self-report scale can identify high expressed emotions and predict higher relapse risk in

schizophrenia. *Comprehensive Psychiatry, 89*, 1-6. doi:10.1016/j.comppsych.2018.12.001

38. Nivard, M. G., Gage, S. H., Hottenga, J. J., Beijsterveldt, C. E., Abdellaoui, A., Bartels, M., . . . Middeldorp, C. M. (2017). Genetic overlap between schizophrenia and developmental psychopathology: Longitudinal and multivariate polygenic risk prediction of common psychiatric traits during development. *Schizophrenia Bulletin, 43*(6), 1197-1207. doi:10.1093/schbul/sbx031

39. Oliver, D., Davies, C., Crossland, G., Lim, S., Gifford, G., Mcguire, P., & Fusar-Poli, P. (2018). Can we reduce the duration of untreated psychosis? A systematic review and meta-analysis of controlled interventional studies. *Schizophrenia Bulletin, 44*(6), 1362-1372. doi:10.1093/schbul/sbx166

40. Ortega-Alonso, A., Ekelund, J., Sarin, A., Miettunen, J., Veijola, J., Järvelin, M., & Hennah, W. (2017). Genome-wide association study of psychosis proneness in the Finnish population. *Schizophrenia Bulletin, 43*(6), 1304-1314. doi:10.1093/schbul/sbx006

41. Poppe, A. B., Barch, D. M., Carter, C. S., Gold, J. M., Ragland, J. D., Silverstein, S. M., & Macdonald, A. W. (2016). Reduced frontoparietal activity in schizophrenia is linked to a specific deficit in goal maintenance: A multisite functional imaging study. *Schizophrenia Bulletin, 42*(5), 1149-1157. doi:10.1093/schbul/sbw036

42. Pries, L., Guloksuz, S., Have, M. T., Graaf, R. D., Dorsselaer, S. V., Gunther, N., . . . Os, J. V. (2018). Evidence that environmental and familial risks for psychosis additively impact a multidimensional subthreshold psychosis syndrome. *Schizophrenia Bulletin, 44*(4), 710-719. doi:10.1093/schbul/sby051

43. Reininghaus, U., Kempton, M. J., Valmaggia, L., Craig, T. K., Garety, P., Onyejiaka, A., . . . Morgan, C. (2016). Stress sensitivity, aberrant salience, and threat anticipation in early psychosis: An experience sampling study. *Schizophrenia Bulletin, 42*(3), 712-722. doi:10.1093/schbul/sbv190

44. Rosenzweig, M. R., Breedlove, S. M., & Watson, N. V. (2005). *Biological Psychology: An Introduction to Behavioral and Cognitive Neuroscience*. Sunderland, MA: Sinauer Associates.

45. Samara, M. T., Nikolakopoulou, A., Salanti, G., & Leucht, S. (2018). How many patients with schizophrenia do not respond to antipsychotic drugs in the short term? An analysis based on individual patient data from randomized controlled trials. *Schizophrenia Bulletin*. doi:10.1093/schbul/sby095

46. Schmidt, A., Cappucciati, M., Radua, J., Rutigliano, G., Rocchetti, M., Dell'Osso, L., . . . Fusar-Poli, P. (2016). Improving prognostic accuracy in subjects at clinical high risk for psychosis: Systematic review of predictive models and meta-analytical sequential testing simulation. *Schizophrenia Bulletin*. doi:10.1093/schbul/sbw098

47. Selten, J., Booij, J., Buwalda, B., & Meyer-Lindenberg, A. (2017). Biological mechanisms whereby social exclusion may contribute to the etiology of psychosis: A narrative review. *Schizophrenia Bulletin*. doi:10.1093/schbul/sbw180

48. Shahab, S., Stefanik, L., Foussias, G., Lai, M., Anderson, K. K., & Voineskos, A. N. (2017). Sex and diffusion tensor imaging of white matter in schizophrenia: A systematic review plus meta-analysis of the corpus callosum. *Schizophrenia Bulletin*, 44(1), 203-221. doi:10.1093/schbul/sbx049

49. Shevlin, M., Mcelroy, E., Bentall, R. P., Reininghaus, U., & Murphy, J. (2016). The psychosis continuum: Testing a bifactor model of psychosis in a general population sample. *Schizophrenia Bulletin*, 43(1), 133-141. doi:10.1093/schbul/sbw067

50. Silverstein, S. M., Spaulding, W. D., & Menditto, A. A. (2006). *Schizophrenia*. Cambridge, MA: Hogrefe & Huber.

51. Sin, J., Gillard, S., Spain, D., Cornelius, V., Chen, T., & Henderson, C. (2017). Effectiveness of psychoeducational interventions for family carers of people with psychosis: A systematic review and meta-analysis. *Clinical Psychology Review*, 56, 13-24. doi:10.1016/j.cpr.2017.05.002

52. Stanfield, A. C., Philip, R. C., Whalley, H., Romaniuk, L., Hall, J., Johnstone, E. C., & Lawrie, S. M. (2017). Dissociation of brain activation in autism and schizotypal personality disorder during social judgments. *Schizophrenia Bulletin*, 43(6), 1220-1228. doi:10.1093/schbul/sbx083

53. Tan, T., Wang, W., Williams, J., Ma, K., Cao, Q., & Yan, Z. (2018). Stress exposure in dopamine D4 receptor knockout mice induces schizophrenia-like behaviors via disruption of GABAergic transmission. *Schizophrenia Bulletin*. doi:10.1093/schbul/sby163

54. Tarrier, N. (2008). Schizophrenia and other psychotic disorders. In *Clinical Handbook of Psychological Disorders: A Step-by-Step Treatment Manual* (4th ed., pp. 463-491). New York: Guilford Press.

55. *The ICD-10 Classification of Mental and Behavioural Disorders: Clinical Descriptions and Diagnostic Guidelines*. (1992). Geneva: World Health Organization.

56. Veling, W., Pot-Kolder, R., Counotte, J., Os, J. V., & Gaag, M. V. (2016). Environmental social stress, paranoia and psychosis liability: A virtual reality study. *Schizophrenia Bulletin*, 42(6), 1363-1371. doi:10.1093/schbul/sbw031

57. Vermeulen, J. M., Rooijen, G. V., Marita P J Van De Kerkhof, Sutterland, A. L., Correll, C. U., & Haan, L. D. (2018). Clozapine and long-term mortality risk in patients with schizophrenia: A systematic review and meta-analysis of studies lasting 1.1–12.5 years. *Schizophrenia Bulletin*, 45(2), 315-329. doi:10.1093/schbul/sby052

58. Wang, A. K., & Miller, B. J. (2017). Meta-analysis of cerebrospinal fluid cytokine and tryptophan catabolite alterations in psychiatric patients: Comparisons between schizophrenia, bipolar disorder, and depression. *Schizophrenia Bulletin*, 44(1), 75-83. doi:10.1093/schbul/sbx035

59. Waters, F., & Fernyhough, C. (2016). Hallucinations: A systematic review of points of similarity and difference across diagnostic

	classes. *Schizophrenia Bulletin, 43*(1), 32-43. doi:10.1093/schbul/sbw132
60.	Wehman, P. (2012). Supported employment: What is it? *Journal of Vocational Rehabilitation, 37*(2), 139-142.
61.	Weisman, O., Guri, Y., Gur, R. E., Mcdonald-Mcginn, D. M., Calkins, M. E., Tang, S. X., . . . Gothelf, D. (2017). Subthreshold psychosis in 22q11.2 deletion syndrome: Multisite naturalistic study. *Schizophrenia Bulletin, 43*(5), 1079-1089. doi:10.1093/schbul/sbx005
62.	Zavos, H. M., Eley, T. C., Mcguire, P., Plomin, R., Cardno, A. G., Freeman, D., & Ronald, A. (2016). Shared etiology of psychotic experiences and depressive symptoms in adolescence: A longitudinal twin study. *Schizophrenia Bulletin, 42*(5), 1197-1206. doi:10.1093/schbul/sbw021
63.	Zhang, J., Lencz, T., Zhang, R. X., Nitta, M., Maayan, L., John, M., . . . Correll, C. U. (2016). Pharmacogenetic associations of antipsychotic drug-related weight gain: A systematic review and meta-analysis. *Schizophrenia Bulletin, 42*(6), 1418-1437. doi:10.1093/schbul/sbw058

Printed in Great Britain
by Amazon